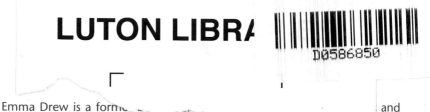
Emma Drew is a forme~ ~ and health projects with charities and the National Healt~ ~~~~~~ ~~ par-ticular interests in equality, social mobility, reading and gender, and how these interact with mental health. She is a Fellow of the Royal Society of Arts and lives in Brighton with her daughter.

Overcoming Common Problems Series

Selected titles

A full list of titles is available from Sheldon Press,
36 Causton Street, London SW1P 4ST and on our website at
www.sheldonpress.co.uk

Breast Cancer: Your treatment choices
Dr Terry Priestman

Chronic Fatigue Syndrome: What you need to know about CFS/ME
Dr Megan A. Arroll

Cider Vinegar
Margaret Hills

Coeliac Disease: What you need to know
Alex Gazzola

Coping Successfully with Hiatus Hernia
Dr Tom Smith

Coping with Difficult Families
Dr Jane McGregor and Tim McGregor

Coping with Epilepsy
Dr Pamela Crawford and Fiona Marshall

Coping with Memory Problems
Dr Sallie Baxendale

Coping with the Psychological Effects of Illness
Dr Fran Smith, Dr Carina Eriksen
and Professor Robert Bor

Coping with Schizophrenia
Professor Kevin Gournay and Debbie Robson

Coping with Thyroid Disease
Mark Greener

Depressive Illness: The curse of the strong
Dr Tim Cantopher

Dr Dawn's Guide to Brain Health
Dr Dawn Harper

Dr Dawn's Guide to Heart Health
Dr Dawn Harper

Dr Dawn's Guide to Weight and Diabetes
Dr Dawn Harper

Dr Dawn's Guide to Women's Health
Dr Dawn Harper

The Empathy Trap: Understanding antisocial personalities
Dr Jane McGregor and Tim McGregor

The Fibromyalgia Healing Diet
Christine Craggs-Hinton

Fibromyalgia: Your treatment guide
Christine Craggs-Hinton

Helping Elderly Relatives
Jill Eckersley

The Holistic Health Handbook
Mark Greener

How to Stop Worrying
Dr Frank Tallis

Invisible Illness: Coping with misunderstood conditions
Dr Megan A. Arroll and Professor
Christine P. Dancey

Living with the Challenges of Dementia: A guide for family and friends
Patrick McCurry

Living with Complicated Grief
Professor Craig A. White

Living with Fibromyalgia
Christine Craggs-Hinton

Living with Hearing Loss
Dr Don McFerran, Lucy Handscomb
and Dr Cherilee Rutherford

Overcoming Fear with Mindfulness
Deborah Ward

Overcoming Low Self-esteem with Mindfulness
Deborah Ward

Overcoming Stress
Professor Robert Bor, Dr Carina Eriksen
and Dr Sara Chaudry

Overcoming Worry and Anxiety
Dr Jerry Kennard

Physical Intelligence: How to take charge of your weight
Dr Tom Smith

Post-Traumatic Stress Disorder: Recovery after accident and disaster
Professor Kevin Gournay

The Self-Esteem Journal
Alison Waines

The Stroke Survival Guide
Mark Greener

Ten Steps to Positive Living
Dr Windy Dryden

Treating Arthritis: The drug-free way
Margaret Hills and Christine Horner

Understanding High Blood Pressure
Dr Shahid Aziz and Dr Zara Aziz

Understanding Yourself and Others: Practical ideas from the world of coaching
Bob Thomson

When Someone You Love Has Depression: A handbook for family and friends
Barbara Baker

Overcoming Common Problems

The Whole Person Recovery Handbook

EMMA DREW

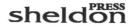

First published in Great Britain in 2015

Sheldon Press
36 Causton Street
London SW1P 4ST
www.sheldonpress.co.uk

British Library Cataloguing-in-Publication Data
A catalogue record for this book is available from the British Library

ISBN 978-1-84709-324-0
eBook ISBN 978-1-84709-325-7

Typeset by Fakenham Prepress Solutions, Fakenham, Norfolk NR21 8NN
First printed in Great Britain by Ashford Colour Press
Subsequently digitally printed in Great Britain

eBook by Fakenham Prepress Solutions, Fakenham, Norfolk NR21 8NN

Produced on paper from sustainable forests

In all evils which admit a remedy, impatience is to be avoided, because it wastes that time and attention in complaints that, if properly applied, might remove the cause.

Samuel Johnson, from The Rambler *32 (Stoicism) (1750)*

Contents

Acknowledgements

This book emerged from my personal encounters with the experiences of hundreds of people – face to face, in books, in broadcast media, at home, at work, at play. It would be impossible to thank everyone who has taught me something, and similarly impossible to ask forgiveness of everyone whom I may have misunderstood. There are however some individuals to whom I am particularly grateful. I must thank all the experts, by experience and by profession, who have contributed to the Royal Society of Arts' Whole Person Recovery work, especially Carley, Brian, Rebecca, Steve and the women who were kind enough to meet with me in Chichester. For tea and encouragement in an unusual environment, thanks to Lady (Doreen) Massey. I continue to be in awe of my interviewees for their humanity, strength and generosity; you know who you are. And I would like to thank Fiona Marshall at Sheldon Press for recognizing that there might be a place in the world for this imperfect but hopeful little book.

Foreword

I was Chair of the National Treatment Agency (England) for 12 years; I visited many drug services and talked to drug users and their families. Some needed more support than others. Some wrestled with poverty, unemployment and deprivation. Some did not. Substance misuse (that is, of drugs, alcohol, tobacco and prescription or over-the-counter drugs) can damage not only individuals but also families, friends and communities. It can rob people of jobs, homes and relationships. Not only can successful drug treatment protect public and personal health, it has been calculated that every £1 spent on drug treatment saves £2.50 in costs to society in terms of health and well-being and crime.

This timely and helpful book is eminently readable, reflective and non-judgemental. It focuses on case studies derived from personal encounters with those who are substance misusers. Emma Drew's book talks of 'real-life recovery', living with the past and finding positive steps forward into self-acceptance. It is not simple. People often work through many relapses and much agony. *The Whole Person Recovery Handbook* discusses managing physical and mental health, skills for life, and gaining identity and self-esteem. It describes various treatment programmes from an objective viewpoint.

There are many ways of treating addiction but, ultimately, the individual has to take charge of his or her own life. We know that the best form of treatment is one that is designed with the individual in mind. Recovering from addiction is personal but can be helped by knowing about the paths others have taken. By providing case studies in this helpful book, Emma gives readers the opportunity to identify with the struggles of others and to find strength in the positive outcomes.

Baroness Massey of Darwen

Introduction
Well, how did I get here?

In 2006 I planted a plum tree in my garden in memory of my friend Mark, who died on his boat in the Sea of Cortez, off the coast of Mexico. As I write, I can see the tree through the window. It has taken well and promises every year to fruit generously, until the pigeons come along and help themselves to the young unripe plums, leaving us none.

Mark would have appreciated the irony. He was a childhood friend with whom I reconnected many times as an adult, a help and support when the practicalities of single parenthood left me juggling frantically and in need of assistance. He was also a recover--ing alcoholic. On his travels around the world he was able to keep going by checking in with a local branch of Alcoholics Anonymous (AA), whether in the UK, the Caribbean, the USA or elsewhere. As a lad I remember him being fiercely critical of his own father's drinking, yet in the end the weight of circumstances (including a debilitating facial injury) overwhelmed him too. AA meetings were not enough. Travel and adventure were not enough.

I was keen for my daughter, as she was growing up, to know that some men can be kind and decent and friendly, to have a male role model, someone who was self-aware and capable. Mark largely fulfilled that role for several years. His loss was devastating, and made me reflect very deeply as to what I had or had not done to help or understand him over the three decades I had known him. Between the ages of 15 and 45, I lost ten friends and colleagues – all male – to suicide, intoxication and excessive risk-taking. I had a lot to think about, including why, when mental health and treatment services were so obviously designed around the needs of men, so many men were still suffering; and why women with the same problems were so likely to end up in the criminal justice system, or having their children taken away, or simply not being helped at all. I was coming across these questions a lot in my professional life, and I felt completely stumped by our collective failure to design services that 'worked'. At the time it was reported that people being treated for addiction on the National Health Service (NHS) had only a 16 per cent chance of being free of alcohol or substance misuse one year after leaving treatment. That's a worse success rate than for most cancer treatments.

My own story

But who am I to be writing this? What qualifies me? In the spirit of openness, I will share a little of my story. There are alcoholics in my family, although only one of them was ever labelled as such (to my knowledge) while I was growing up. My grandmother was in many respects a remarkable woman. Was she 'self-medicating'? Certainly. She had lost a brother in the war and a child in a terrible accident a few years later. My limited understanding of what happened after that does not offer a positive impression of the professional psychological help she was offered at the time. This was the 1950s, after all.

Her relationship with my mother was fraught. My mother went on to suffer her own demons, and married very young. She and my father coped badly with their large family and low income, and in addition my father's work – he was a policeman – regularly took him into traumatic situations for which the usual solution was to go to the pub afterwards. Anger, drunkenness and violence were commonplace with both parties. So my childhood was shaped by the reverberations of traumatic events that happened to other people. That meant that I became familiar with, and to some degree came to accept, the behaviour that can go with a vortex of trauma, distress and addiction that pulls everyone in: emotional-rollercoaster parenting, manipulation and bullying, resentment (addiction and resentment go hand in hand), lies, financial pressures, arguments, fractured personalities, and indeed in our case violence.

My friendships outside home sustained me through this. Later, however, as a young adult, I became aware that alcohol and 'recreational' drug use had become normal for me – as it was and is for a lot of people. I spent time with artists, writers, musicians, in a lively and exciting world where drugs and alcohol were normalized – though I would not want to stereotype those professions; a doctor, lawyer, teacher, geneticist, builder, stay-at-home mother, member of the House of Lords, company executive or van driver is just as likely to abuse alcohol and drugs as anybody else.

I became aware of what I was doing and that I did not want to follow the addict's path, so I made a conscious decision not to. I moderated my intake, avoided the more dangerous drugs and had periods of abstinence from alcohol through choice. It took some effort. But I was still accepting of certain types of behaviour that for other people might ring alarm bells. Some time later I met a man called Chris, who became my partner. Kind, decent, friendly, approved of by most of my friends. I use the word 'most' advisedly, because there was one person who raised a doubt that I only came to understand much later. The plausibility of the addict means that perfectly capable people find themselves being taken in. The following little sketch barely touches upon the depth of the trauma we went through, but it gives an idea, I hope, of why I am keen to share my learning with others.

I had been involved for some years with the Royal Society of Arts (RSA) in London, so when an article appeared in the *RSA Journal* saying that the society was launching a pilot 'whole person recovery' project, I was enthusiastic.[1] I was particularly keen to see two things happen: for people to be involved in creating their own pathways to recovery from mental suffering, and for the whole of their lives and circumstances to be taken into account in their treatment. I knew from a project I had worked on that for women the issues of financial independence and safe, trustworthy and affordable childcare were important for *any* kind of quality of life, so for women in recovery it seemed to me doubly vital that these challenges should be addressed effectively. At that point I still had shocks to come as to how bad things could get for some women. But I did have the professional skills to help women who felt themselves to be more or less unemployable to set themselves up in social enterprises, volunteering or self-employment, so I offered to become involved in the RSA's work.

For years too I had spent many drunken evenings sharing both banter and stories of mental anguish with male friends, so I wanted to understand why when some men were prepared to talk to me, an unqualified and wayward friend, about what was going on in their heads, they would not seek help from people far better able to provide it. Chris freely shared with me his experiences of anxiety, but I later learned that was only the tip of the iceberg. My alarm bells did not ring.

As I talked to Chris about what was happening with the RSA's work, he became more and more supportive. He liked a drink (at that point I had no idea how much, nor what else he liked), and he had been a bit of a party animal when younger, so he knew some of the territory, I felt. He had become in middle age a respectable project manager for a major company, with a degree in architecture and responsibility for people's lives and safety on construction sites. He had a middle-class accent, was quite well read and had a very good income. He played classical guitar and was absurdly affectionate, both to me and to his children from a previous relationship. I felt lucky to have met him. What I did not know was that he was engaged in a battle to the death with inner demons that in the end would nearly destroy us both. Three years after meeting him, in order to save my daughter and myself, I had to ask him to leave. Three months later, having suffered a heart attack induced by years of cocaine abuse, he was dead.

The right kind of help came, but too little too late. The wrong kind came too soon in Chris's life and blocked out the light. People covered up for him. They paid his debts (except the money he owed me). They excused his behaviour. They told him his behaviour was not as bad as it was. They joined in the drinking, drug taking and gambling, about which I was largely ignorant until it was too late. People forgave Chris unspeakable acts of cruelty and deceit, accepted his excuses and manipulations. They told lies on his behalf. There was a right royal maelstrom of stories and deceptions, in fact. When things went wrong *it was always somebody else's fault*. Finally, the effort of holding these narratives together, of keeping the truth hidden and of the constantly repeated self-medication, caused Chris to lose his mind. He developed drug-induced psychosis and became a monster. The addict controlled the man.

As someone who had seen substance abuse close up, and who had worked as a volunteer on a recovery project for three years, you would think that I would have noticed that my partner had a problem with drugs and alcohol. But I didn't. He liked a trip to the pub, but I live in Brighton, a city known for its party atmosphere. I knew he suffered, as many people do, with anxiety, but it wasn't until six months before his death that he finally started to come clean, so to speak, about the full extent of the problem, by which time it was much too late for his physical health. He was also up to his ears in debt, as it turned out, and compulsively borrowed more and more, financially abusing me in order to feed his addictions.

Before his death Chris had a (too brief) spell in a Priory rehabilitation clinic, where his was described by his therapist as 'the worst case of cross-addiction' he had seen. Cross-addiction is where someone's addictive behaviour is transferred from one substance or behaviour to another in a desperate search for gratification and oblivion. In Chris's case this meant cocaine, heroin, alcohol, cigarettes, codeine (an over-the-counter painkiller), diazepam (a prescription sedative) and gambling. And that's just what I know about. On the afternoon before his admission to the Priory he consumed an unknown amount of heroin, 84 codeine tablets, eight cans of super-strong lager and most of a bottle of brandy. He probably smoked about 40 cigarettes that day too. He was intercepted by the police three times. A complete stranger half his size had to pull him out of the way of a bus (whoever you were, thank you).

I was almost bankrupted by Chris's behaviour in the time we were together. Yet although what happened to me might fit the legal definition of certain criminal acts – 'obtaining pecuniary advantage by deception', say, 'false imprisonment' and 'threatening behaviour', I was unable to have those events recorded as crimes by the police, despite reporting them at the time and later.

Chris's rationalizations were highly plausible. When in his most psychotic state the police attended to him, they were calm and well-trained, for which I shall always be grateful, but the truth is that when someone is being terrorized in their own home by a person who has lost his or her mind to addiction, the police need to act more decisively. Famously, many addicts will not address their problem until they reach 'rock bottom' – in my case I felt that the failure of the police to 'section'[2] my partner and put him in a place of safety (I ended up having to pay for him to go to a hotel) amounted to forcing me to collude in his addiction. With hindsight, I recognize that this was first-hand experience of an unfortunately widespread police response to male aggression that leaves the victim to make a decision about the detention or prosecution of the perpetrator, notwithstanding that making such a decision can put a person at further risk and that in the context of other crimes the police do seem to make their own decisions about whether to take action.

Chris's addiction up until that point had commandeered all of his wit, empathy and intelligence in order to conceal his habits and fool me, along with his employer and plenty of other people. Perhaps you think I didn't challenge his behaviour? As a matter of fact I did, regularly, but one should never underestimate the fiendish resourcefulness of addiction, not to mention the plausibility of the addict in its grip. Addiction destroys loving relationships precisely because it destroys trust.

Chris had been an addict for 25 years. Maybe, you would think, his family or ex-wife might have told me what they knew about his history and the threat he posed to my daughter and me? Well, no. In effect, middle-class 'niceness' and family collusion allowed him to become far more ill than many poorer people who end up in worse circumstances. The business of 'enabling' addiction and 'co-dependency' is also something we will touch on in this book, and there are lots of helpful guides and websites out there that can help you understand better how not to make things worse by encouraging your own or someone else's addictive behaviour, inadvertently or otherwise. Breaking co-dependency is painful and people will often need support. Some helpful references and places to go are listed in the 'Helpful organizations' section at the back of the book.

I was lucky. I am able to move forward, step by step. I am fit, well and have had an interesting and varied career. My relationship with my daughter is warm and loving; I enjoy a happy and peaceful home life. Many of the people I knew through work and social-izing were not so fortunate. When I mentioned, in a talk at the RSA in London in 2010, the number of friends I had lost to addiction and related conditions, the intake of breath from the audience was audible. It needs saying repeatedly: people are dying in large numbers. Addiction is an epidemic. Treatment is not working for many. Thinking seriously about how to make recovery work is no longer a dry policy debate but an urgent matter of how to reduce very costly, widespread distress and prevent suffering and thou-sands of deaths, including those of some of our most creative and intelligent people. So, in a sense, this book is for my friends, whom I still miss and for whom I wish the world had not been such a harsh and intolerable place.

For me, learning about other people's recovery came together with learning – rather later than you might expect – what it might mean for myself. It took a long time to recover my sense of balance, and rebuilding our lives is a work in progress. Understanding that the delusions can take in more than one person is important, because the potential solutions are also likely to involve more than addicts themselves, and are likely to entail little steps forward (and setbacks) rather than the simple straight line to perfect health that is so often promised by 'treatment' but so rarely materializes. For every person who is directly addicted, it is estimated that a further nine people are being affected, some of them wittingly or unwittingly colluding in the problem. My message for people helping others with addiction is: look after yourself and make no assumptions. Seek support from people with knowledge and experience, whether professional or personal. Read as much as you can.

Paths to well-being

As we shall see, addiction has some very particular characteristics (the 'Helpful organizations' section at the back of the book will help you find more information). But very often addiction is rooted in early or long-term suffering that may have led to other problems like anxiety and depression, compulsive behaviour or difficulties with anger. Contrary to popular myth, there is no neat boundary between addiction and other forms of mental distress. So this book will focus not on the problem – there are already lots of places to find out about that – but on paths towards health and well-being that have been tried and tested by others.

In the face of problems such as those faced by Chris, AA meetings were never going to be enough. The AA line that addiction is a disease (or sometimes 'dis-ease') can be helpful to a point, it seems to me, because it helps explain how little control a person might have over what is happening. However, it is logically inconsistent that a disease, which is a medical definition, can be entirely 'cured' by the moral and spiritual lessons of the AA fellowship. Meetings are powerfully important for many of AA's participants, but for people like Chris – not religious and indeed probably harmed by a religious upbringing – making oneself vulnerable and surrendering to a 'higher power' or idea of God in a public forum feels anti-intuitive, dangerous even. I should be clear that I recognize the vital role that both AA and Narcotics Anonymous (NA) play in the lives of many people in recovery from addiction, not to mention the support provided to family and friends through the related organization Al-Anon. What I am arguing though is that for *some* people these are *not enough*, and for some they are *not right*.

For me mental suffering and self-medication are the product of people's entire life experience. They are complex and wrapped up in who we are as people, whether we regard ourselves as 'ill' or not. Until we learn to see the whole person, we will never have recovery services that work.

So this book is for people in recovery, for people thinking about it, for family members, friends and supporters. It is for people in health, social services, the charity sector and education who would like to understand a little more about addiction, mental suffering and recovery, and what you can do to help. It offers an overview of some humane ways that people are finding to improve their lives. Its particular focus is on recovery from addiction, but it is not only about that, and I hope anyone who has an interest in recovery from mental health difficulties may find something in here to enlighten or inspire them.

Most of all it is the product of shared stories and real lived experiences. We will look in detail at how people have experienced the hold and struggle of addiction and illness; at the differences between treatment or 'medical' recovery and 'whole person' or 'person-centred' recovery; and at the ideas, techniques, forms of support and ways of being that people have used to help themselves. Throughout the book you will find quotes from people I have interviewed, participants at conferences and training events, and other first-person testimony from published sources of people in recovery or who are part of the recovery journey in some other way: family, friends, partners, health professionals, volunteers or support workers. Everyone is anonymous. The point of these quotes is that they are from real life, from people who have experienced recovery and have a story to tell.

1

Same as it ever was: experiences of addiction and treatment

'No one chooses to become a victim of the system.'

(Volunteer, Whole Person Recovery project,
Royal Society of Arts Journal, 2010)

'These systems are for us. If the system doesn't work, we have to get rid of it.'

(Russell Brand, *Stop the War on Drugs*,
BBC Television, 15 December 2014)

If you are reading this then the chances are that you, or someone you know, has a problem with health, behaviour or both that is causing difficulties. You may be in some distress. Maybe it is part of your job to help someone else. Maybe someone in your family or circle of friends is in trouble. Very likely you would like some ideas about how to change things for the better. If so, this book is for you: it is based on the lives of people who have had experiences like yours, and have decided to share their stories of recovery. For some, addiction has been the key problem. For others, misusing alcohol, street drugs, prescription medicines or gambling (or a combination of these) is one part of a larger picture of mental health or life struggles. For yet others, addiction is not the main issue at all. The point is that the principles of successful recovery are the same, even if the day-to-day experiences of it are as varied as the people involved.

Addiction and society

Think of a typical evening out: perhaps a show or a concert; a trip to the pub; a dinner with friends or family. Now try to think of the same event without the alcohol (or dope, or diazepam). For a very few people, the event will be the same. For most, we are talking about a very different occasion, or even an impossibility. In the UK today, for many people, it is normal to drink alcohol most days.

The substances of intoxication, recreation and medication are all around us, pretty much all of the time, from the top to the bottom of society. With them, the codes of behaviour they attract, which we often learn as young people, become social norms. The altered state that these substances create may be temporary and benign. Or it may not. To be lifted out of mental distress for a short time, even if you were not particularly aware of those underlying feelings, is deeply seductive and can feel liberating. And as we will hear, chasing that first-time feeling of freedom and delight can be what drives addiction. People's routes into addiction are different, and what you will *not* find here is moral judgement about how that happened. It can and does happen to anybody.

> Drugs are amazing. They take you to a dimension you've never been to.[1]

> A lot of people [drink or take drugs] to self-medicate: drink's a symptom of what's going on – you can have such powerful emotions. It's so easy to take these chemicals to take it all away again.[2]

The musician Goldie described his relationship with drugs as dealing with 'a massive emotional hole in my life'.

Even when someone identifies that they have a problem with reliance on alcohol, street drugs or prescription medicines, moving away from that into successful recovery can be very, very difficult, as anyone who has tried it will tell you. But it can be done. The people in this book prove it and my aim is to share their insights and offer hope.

Addictive thinking

Let's begin, though, by taking a brief look at the nature of addiction. Figures suggest that 1 in 10 of the adult UK population experiences addiction. When nicotine and prescription drugs are taken into account, it may be as many as 1 in 4 or 1 in 3. Stigma, shame and the very nature of the condition make it hard to acknowledge, diagnose and treat successfully. How do you recover from a condition that you don't think you have?

There are few better descriptions of how addicts think than a standard work that is often issued (prescribed, as it were) to patients on addiction treatment programmes at the Priory Hospitals:

Abraham Twerski's *Addictive Thinking: Understanding Self-Deception*.[3]
It gives a clear explanation of the thought patterns and behaviours
that make addiction so painful to live with and so difficult to treat.
Twerski is also helpful on the severity of the condition and the
confusion caused by it: 'Sometimes people with addictive diseases
are misdiagnosed as schizophrenic. They may have some of the
same symptoms, including delusions, hallucinations, inappropriate
moods, very abnormal behaviour.'[4]

Here are some quick definitions of the typical characteristics of
addictive thinking:

> *Denial*: this does not mean telling lies. It is a way of rejecting
> the reality that is 'neither conscious nor wilful, and the addict
> may sincerely believe they are telling the truth'.[5]

> *Rationalization*: this means 'offering good, that is plausible,
> reasons. That does not mean that all rationalizations are good
> reasons . . . [they] divert attention from true reasons. They
> not only divert others' attention from the truth, but also the
> addict's.'[6]

> *Projection*: 'placing the blame on others for things we are really
> responsible for ourselves'.[7]

> *Co-dependency*: 'A co-dependent person is one who has let
> another's behaviour affect him or her, and who is obsessed with
> controlling that person's behaviour.'[8]

For the purposes of this book I will assume readers have some
basic familiarity with those ideas, such as how people will find
an apparently plausible rationalization for their addiction (or the
bad behaviour arising from it), such as real physical pain, a broken
heart, a terrible job, a lack of positive choices. Twerski is brisk
and to the point, perhaps some would say insufficiently compassionate, but he writes with great knowledge. This description was
very familiar to me: 'Blaming someone else seems to relieve an
addict from the responsibility of making changes: "As long as
you do this to me, you cannot expect me to change." Since the
others are not likely to change, the drinking and other drug use
can continue.'[9]

William Burroughs, the renowned (or notorious) writer, puts
things from the addict's point of view:

'A dope fiend is a man in total need of dope. Beyond a certain frequency need knows absolutely no limit or control. In the words of total need: "*Wouldn't you?*" Yes you would. You would lie, cheat, inform on your friends, steal, do *anything* to satisfy total need.'[10]

Author Miranda Critchley, who quotes Burroughs above, goes on to say that his 'total belief in the possibility of a cure added to the force of his writing, as did the responsibility he felt to publicise addiction treatments and campaign for better care'.

Myths about addiction and recovery

Denial is one of the cruellest, most harmful and most slippery aspects of addiction to manage, and this is where thinking about 'recovery' rather than 'treatment' shows its strength. But in order to get to grips with how recovery is different from treatment, we need first to deal briefly with a couple of common myths.

First of these is the suggestion that alcoholism is a death sentence. Figures from a study of 43,000 adults by the National Institute of Alcohol Abuse and Alcoholism cited by Stanton Peele, an established writer on addiction in the USA, suggest that 'Remission is commonplace: in the long run, about three-quarters of alcoholics achieve full recovery. Of this sizeable majority, "about 75% of persons who recover from alcohol dependence do so without seeking any kind of help".'[11] Peele specifically urges caution in relation to neurobiological models of addiction and medicalized treatment, seeing these as promoting the interests of a privatized American healthcare system rather than the interests of the addict. He argues that 'our best data . . . show that addiction should be de-medicalized in favour of a model that encourages the advancement of psychological and environmental conditions that naturally prevent and dispel addiction'.

Second is the belief that heroin is automatically and permanently addictive. Will people always be defeated by the horrors of withdrawal? Here are the views of literary academic and recovering addict Michael Clune, quoted by Miranda Critchley in the *London Review of Books*:

Clune himself downplays the effects of withdrawal – 'the sad truth is that the physical symptoms of withdrawal really aren't so terrible. If you've ever had a bad case of the flu, you basically know what the physical symptoms are like' – and disagrees with [William] Burroughs that anyone who uses heroin will automatically get addicted, an error he thinks 'flows from the common mistake of equating addiction to the drug with the physical dependence that is one of its less pleasant side effects'. His comments on the treatment available for addicts are understated: 'We work with what we have. And I'm profoundly grateful for it.'[12]

So experiences of addiction are varied, and experiences of recovery are equally varied. There are though widely shared patterns of behaviour from which it is possible to learn. A few weeks after my partner Chris came out of rehab, and three months before he died, he went through something that seemed to me worse than the first stages of physical withdrawal, and I wish I had had prior knowledge that it might occur. I was completely unprepared for the crash in mood and behaviour that ultimately led to Chris leaving our flat for good. This second stage of withdrawal is sometimes called 'post-acute withdrawal syndrome' or PAWS. I found it positively frightening and felt entirely unable to deal with the implacable, aggressive and wholly uncommunicative presence that appeared in the midst of our home.[13]

Treatment and recovery: some differences

Here is how Sussex NHS Partnership Trust, a mental health trust delivering services in the south of England, defines the differences between a top-down medical approach to treatment and something more like person-centred recovery. First, 'treatment':

> Up until quite recently, the most common understanding . . . was a medical one that placed the most weight on curing or reducing symptoms. This understanding is still very important and meaningful to caregivers and people who experience mental health difficulties . . . [It] can reduce feelings of self-blame by offering an explanation and treatment options aimed at reducing or managing symptoms. As with a faulty engine, specialist knowledge is required to diagnose and fix the fault.[14]

Now, 'recovery':

> a process of growing beyond the experience of mental health issues and recovering some of the losses that living with mental

distress incurs. For some it's about discovering new opportunities and experiential gains; in these cases great weight is placed upon the social and/or personal aspects of life, depending on what holds most value for the person.

That is, recovery is about slow, careful and profound changes, about finding and building on the positive aspects of life, about working with what you have rather than what you have not, about accepting that imperfection and failure are normal parts of life and learning to get better. Recovery can be seen as a personal journey, and as something that happens in groups, places and networks where people can find empathy and support: 'recovery communities'.

Here is what Al-Anon Family Groups say in their leaflet *Alcoholism: A Merry-Go-Round Named Denial*:

> Act One: The play opens with the alcoholic stating that no one can tell him what to do; he tells them . . .
>
> A planned recovery from alcoholism must begin with the person in the second act. They must learn how people affect each other in this illness and then learn the most difficult part – *that of acting in an entirely different fashion.*
>
> (emphasis original)

At a conference at the Brighton Festival Fringe in 2014 I asked participants to define what recovery meant to them. A health professional came up with: 'Recovery happens to everyone, all the time.' That is, our own natural healing process, when given time, space and the right conditions, is what will drive improvements to our health and well-being. That process may be assisted by other forms of support such as medical treatment, or loving care from friends, or psychotherapy, but the point is that it comes from a person's own natural resources and is self-managed (with help, if that is what a person chooses). The person in recovery takes an increasing amount of responsibility at a pace that works for him or her. It is not *imposed* from an external source such as a time-limited pharmaceutical treatment programme, although of course you may find such programmes helpful and may appreciate being invited to participate. But forcing someone to jump through a series of hoops when he or she is already suffering and failing to cope is often doomed to failure and produces nothing but frustration (and worse) for everyone involved.

Recovery works with the innate ability of the self, in the right circumstances, to heal. This ability, labelled the 'actualizing tendency' by psychologist Carl Rogers (who we will meet again later), can be described as

> a human's basic drive to maintain, develop and enhance their functioning. In a sense it is a fundamental 'life force' that does not abate but constantly urges the person towards development. The actualizing tendency drives the person to make the best they can of their circumstances.[15]

If someone feels broken, damaged, hurt, thwarted by life, then a key is to create the environment in which that person's natural tendency to heal can get to work. This entails looking at the whole person, living in the real world, and trying to find ways to make his or her life not just bearable but something better.

Addiction as disease

It is acceptable in some quarters to view addiction as a disease rather than a self-induced problem – although perhaps not in some of our tabloid newspapers, where the demonization of addicts continues apace, and no doubt the long historical association between journalism and alcohol is alive and well. I say this as someone whose uncle worked on the *News of the World*. People, including addicts, need to know how to protect themselves from the damaging behaviour brought on by addiction, in the way that my daughter and I needed protecting from Chris as he became more ill and dangerous to himself and others – and to do that we need to have a much better shared understanding of the problem.

The difficulty with the disease model of addiction is that while it helps to convey the idea that addiction is a mental health problem and may not be the fault of the addict, which is vital, it also implies that there is a course of 'treatment' that will work in the same way as, say, treatment for a physical problem like gout or head lice. Disappointing experiences of treatment for addiction or indeed other mental health issues can compound a rock-bottom sense of worthlessness that is excruciatingly painful and leads some people back to their old health-destroying habits. There is a further complication: if we criminalize addicts, as increasingly seems to be happening as I write, with one local authority seeking to prosecute the mother of a baby born with foetal alcohol syndrome, then a supposedly criminal act is logically a matter for the criminal justice system, and cannot also be primarily an issue for the health service to address. If someone's addictive behaviour is rooted in profound feelings of self-hatred and worthlessness, sending them to prison and telling them they are bad and worthless is not likely to be helpful. Criminalizing addiction has filled our prisons to bursting with people who are most unlikely to be in a position to deal with their psychological difficulties, and who therefore are on course to re-offend upon release. It is a most expensive, cruel and largely pointless way of (not) tackling the problem.

> I was living in a bail hostel and there were 49 men in there and me and I was really harassed in there. They ran a book, the first night I stayed there, they ran a book on who was going to sleep with me first. And they knew I was a valium addict. One of them knocked on my door, gave me £20 in valium and I woke up the next day with him in the bed next to me . . . So he won £30 cos they'd all put a quid in. I had to stay there. It was a homeless shelter.[16]

People who want to conceal their addiction will use every ounce of ingenuity they have to do so. They don't want to be caught, after all. The chances are that they already hate themselves for what they do, and feel ashamed. In many cases facing the pain caused by their addictive behaviour is simply too much to bear, so they seek to blot out those thoughts with denial, drink or drugs and the cycle of addiction is prolonged. Such people may seek to deflect blame on to others. The range of excuses we humans can create for ourselves when we feel bad about something we have done is immense at the best of times – addicts turn that into an art form.

The hardest lesson for me to learn was not to be angry with the addict. Anger is a sane and reasonable response to being deliberately hurt, or having your money stolen, or being deceived or humiliated. But, crucially, it will not make the addict stop being an addict. *It simply will not work.* One piece of advice I was given that I found helpful when it came to the number one priority of keeping myself and my daughter safe in our home was 'detach but do not abandon'. You cannot fix someone else – only they can do that – but you can be part of the solution rather than part of the problem.

And first of all you can do so by looking after yourself. You and the addict in your life need to be listened to.

> I opened up to someone I didn't know very well and it allowed something to click like a wake-up call.[17]

> Just someone asking the question, 'What's wrong?'

> I started making things up just to go to the doctor. I felt better as soon as I got there.

Experts by profession and experts by experience

The Royal Society of Arts (RSA) developed its pioneering research into drugs, addiction and recovery on the back of a simple but essential assumption: successful recovery requires an *equal* partnership between 'experts by profession' – doctors, therapists, drugs workers, nurses, pharmacists – and 'experts by experience', people with lived experience of addiction and its social, psychological and practical effects, and of other mental health difficulties, and who are, indeed, the experts on their own lives. As we will see, this assumption has pretty radical implications, for the simple reason that it moves power away from professionals and into the hands of people who traditionally may be seen in some quarters as difficult, destructive and untrustworthy.

In other words, if you are a person affected by reliance on addictive behaviour, you are also a decision-maker about your own life and have the support of a team of experts. You may feel vulnerable at this moment, or not ready to take on that role just yet. That is fine. The recovery journey is designed around you, by you, with support. You go at whatever pace and in whatever direction works for you. Relapse is possible. It is not the end of the world. You can learn each time and carry on, if you feel able. You may wish for certain types of treatment as part of what happens, but this is not 'treatment'. It is much bigger than that. And altogether more enjoyable.

The road to recovery

No one, though, should assume recovery is easy. How difficult it might be is hard to understand if you have never had to deal with it. Catherine Amey has written a groundbreaking book about her experiences of psychosis and the mental health system, which is now being used to train social workers wanting to specialize in mental health:

> Treading the path of recovery for me was as excruciating as walking through treacle or over a bed of nails. For a long while I was unable to process the indigestible trauma. After leaving hospital I could not bear to be alone and had a childlike fear of the dark. This lasted for many months. I felt suicidal a lot of the time, even though I had the full support of my husband's family and most of my friends, many of whom carried hope for me when I couldn't carry it for myself. Perversely, it was also a creative time when I drafted many poems and stories for my son.[18]

Amey's book was lent to me by a social worker who also happened to be a neighbour. I was pleased to see how real people's lived experiences were being used to support training in social services because when I went to Foyle's, the UK's largest bookshop, to see what was being recommended to medical students to read and learn about recovery, there was virtually nothing in the textbooks. There was some very brief introductory material on addiction and other mental health problems, but almost nothing on the recovery movement at all. Even the specialist mental health texts had a strong focus on 'treatment', often pharmacological treatment, at the expense of other approaches such as psychotherapy and peer support. So basic training for our doctors and nurses seems barely to touch upon one of the biggest health problems affecting society, nor upon the growing body of evidence suggesting that person-centred recovery is both more effective and more cost-effective than conventional medical treatment programmes.

2

Into the blue again: the growth of the recovery movement

All is not lost, however. There are signs of change. In July 2010, as a result of my involvement with the RSA's Whole Person Recovery project, I was invited to tea in the House of Lords with Lady Doreen Massey, then chair of the National Treatment Agency, the department of the National Health Service (NHS) that dealt with addiction treatment programmes. What I heard there was interested and empathetic support for new approaches, particularly in connection with the predicament faced by women 'service users' in a system designed for and largely run by men.

Earlier in the year I had attended a conference that brought together people in recovery with interested professionals and RSA staff (experts by experience and experts by profession), at which the health experts and policy wonks were able to listen directly to the experiences of people who had sought help from the NHS or their local Drug and Alcohol Action Team (DAAT). Not all of it was terribly flattering to our service providers, and some of the stories were distressing, such as that of the woman who was denied residential rehab support because she was a single mum and had no childcare for while she was away, and who was frightened of losing her children to the care of social services. To this day I treasure the memory of the young lad, 18 or so and used to drinking several litres of cider a day, who made thoughtful and considered but highly critical comments to John McCracken, senior civil servant at the Department of Health. It was not the kind of conversation you witness every day, and it is to the RSA's credit that these two were able to participate on (more or less) equal terms.

This was a key moment at which those currently holding the power and the purse strings were able to listen and take steps to accelerate the process of positive change to care services, to make them more fit for purpose and better able to help the people who need it (not to mention use public resources more effectively). But just as recovery can be two steps forward, one step back, so can change in public services. Power has its own addictive qualities. In any situation where change involves the transfer of power and control, there will be people who do not want to let go. And even while changes are afoot in the way that the health and police services understand how substance misuse and mental health can be managed, the politicians and the press still have a long way to go before overall public perceptions can be substantially changed. And there are vested interests that benefit from the status quo, of course. Which is another reason why recovery and change take courage and support – and kindness.

From treatment to recovery

Public opinion appears to be ahead of the policy makers on this subject. According to research reported by the charity Drugscope, 77 per cent of people agree that investment in drugs treatment programmes is a sensible use of government money, 80 per cent agree that people can become addicted to drugs because of other problems in their lives, and 88 per cent agree that treatment should be available to anybody with a drugs problem who is prepared to address it.[1]

The shift away from 'top down' and directive approaches to 'treatment' towards collaboration between experts by experience and experts by profession inevitably happens at a different rate in different places. The Sussex Partnership NHS Foundation Trust, a teaching trust of the Brighton and Sussex Medical School, is evolving its strategy along these lines. It might not be for everyone, but if you are the kind of person who would find it beneficial to have active involvement and a serious voice and role to play in the design of mental health research or services, you might find this encouraging. For example, the Lived Experience Advisory Forum is founded on the idea of critical friendship – a trusted source of insight, knowledge and experience that can give honest and if necessary critical commentary. The forum entails 'collaboration and consultation in which different and equally valued perspectives join hands in a shared learning journey with the shared goal of improving the quality of research and [its] translation into practice'.[2] At the time of writing the Trust had established groups to look at dementia, psychosis, early interventions in psychosis, mood and anxiety, learning disabilities, substance misuse and neurobehavioural questions. This seems to me like significant progress, especially when you consider the prevalence of mental health conditions in society:

- There were 1.747 million people in contact with specialist mental health services in 2013–14; 105,270 (6 per cent) spent time in hospital.
- There were 21.706 million outpatient and community contacts arranged for mental health service users in 2013–14.
- 53,176 people were detained ('sectioned') under the Mental Health Act in 2013–14.[3]

This, meanwhile, is from guidance for doctors issued by the National Institute for Health and Care Excellence, which provides the formal framework for diagnosis and treatment options paid for by the state:

In the UK, it is estimated that 24% of adults drink in a hazardous or harmful way . . . Levels of self-reported hazardous and harmful drinking are lowest in the central and eastern regions of England (21–24% of men and 10–14% of women). They are highest in the North East, North West and Yorkshire and Humber (26–28% of men, 16–18% of women). Hazardous and harmful drinking are commonly encountered among hospital attendees; approximately 20% of patients admitted to hospital for illnesses unrelated to alcohol are drinking at potentially hazardous levels.[4]

The fact that only 11 per cent of the NHS budget is allocated to mental health services is increasingly the subject of press and public discussion. Not a moment too soon. See this for example:

Sue Bailey, president of the Royal College of Psychiatrists, said: 'Much has been done to improve mental health in the last 10 years but it still does not receive the same attention as physical health, and the consequences can be serious.

'People with severe mental illness have a reduced life expectancy of 15–20 years, yet the majority of reasons for this are avoidable.' . . .

Mental health accounts for 22.8 per cent of the so-called 'disease burden' in the UK – more than cardiovascular disease (16.2 per cent) or cancer (15.9 per cent).[5]

Inevitably there is resistance in some quarters to allocating a greater share of public resources to mental health, including among politicians who make choices about public spending priorities: 'The most recently published national surveys of investment for mental

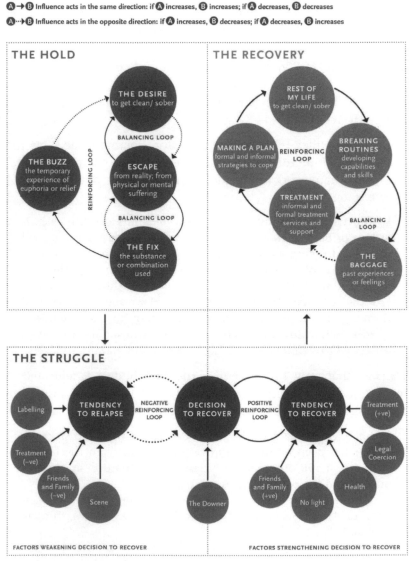

Figure 1 Map of whole person recovery

Reproduced by kind permission of the RSA

health found there had been real terms reductions of 1 per cent for working age adults and 3.1 per cent for older people in 2011/12.'[6] Yet as some of the respondents to the RSA's research into the lives of recovering heroin users show, physical health problems are very often a manifestation of problematic substance use. And by the same token, mental health problems including depressive states and addiction can arise as a consequence of physical health issues.

This emphasizes again how important it is, if recovery is to be effective, to look at the whole of a person's life and circumstances rather than just the symptoms of addiction.

The RSA's Whole Person Recovery project sought to understand in a holistic way how problematic drug and alcohol users become trapped in cycles of addiction, what helps or hinders their journey to recovery, and how their recovery can be sustained. As part of mapping this 'system', they recorded the stories of many individuals and how these related to key elements of the addictive cycle: the Hold, the Struggle and the Recovery (see Figure 1 on p. 14). 'Sam' describes how he was always chasing the 'buzz' of heroin after first using it:

> 'At first it wraps you up in cotton wool . . . but after a month, maybe six weeks, then that hit, all it does is bring you back to normal. You get so ill that you're using as medication.' As Sam's need to seek an Escape from the painful 'rattle' he experienced if he did not use heroin increased, the likelihood of him seeking the Fix increased, which resulted in the Buzz and decreased his immediate desire to Escape. The temporary euphoria and relief of the Buzz also reduced his desire to seek a fundamental solution (the Desire) and get clean. This maintained his involvement in the Hold.[7]

Definitions of abuse and dependence

Conventional medical thinking on addiction, even in recently updated form, differs substantially from the findings of the RSA and others on what effective recovery is and how it is achieved. The American Psychiatric Association publishes *The Diagnostic and Statistical Manual of Mental Disorders*, which has been recently published in its fifth edition (*DSM-V*).[8] This is the standard US desk reference for doctors on all matters to do with mental health, and it is internationally influential. Here is a summary of the *DSM-V* definition of 'substance use disorder':

Substance use disorder in DSM-5 combines the DSM-IV categories of substance abuse and substance dependence into a single disorder measured on a continuum from mild to severe. Each specific substance (other than caffeine, which cannot be diagnosed as a substance use disorder) is addressed as a separate use disorder (e.g., alcohol use disorder, stimulant use disorder, etc.), but nearly all substances are diagnosed based on the same overarching criteria. In this overarching disorder, the criteria have not only been combined, but strengthened. Whereas a diagnosis of substance abuse previously required only one symptom, mild substance use disorder in DSM-5 requires two to three symptoms from a list of 11. Drug craving will be added to the list, and problems with law enforcement will be eliminated because of cultural considerations that make the criteria difficult to apply internationally.

In DSM-IV, the distinction between abuse and dependence was based on the concept of abuse as a mild or early phase and dependence as the more severe manifestation. In practice, the abuse criteria were sometimes quite severe. The revised substance use disorder, a single diagnosis, will better match the symptoms that patients experience.[9]

There are lots of helpful websites that explain how doctors understand addictive disorders using the *DSM-V* criteria, and how they distinguish these from other forms of mental distress. Here is an example:

Substance use disorders span a wide variety of problems arising from substance use, and cover 11 different criteria:

1 TAKING the substance in larger amounts or for longer than you meant to
2 Wanting to cut down or stop using the substance but not managing to
3 Spending a lot of time getting, using, or recovering from use of the substance
4 Cravings and urges to use the substance
5 Not managing to do what you should at work, home or school, because of substance use
6 Continuing to use, even when it causes problems in relationships

7   Giving up important social, occupational or recreational activities because of substance use

8   Using substances again and again, even when it puts you in danger

9   Continuing to use, even when you know you have a physical or psychological problem that could have been caused or made worse by the substance

10 Needing more of the substance to get the effect you want (tolerance)

11 Development of withdrawal symptoms, which can be relieved by taking more of the substance.[10]

You could replace the word 'substance' with the word 'gambling' to see how addictive behaviour and the need to get a fix can take multiple forms. The 'high' comes to replace other, less comfortable feelings that a person wants to get rid of, whether consciously or unconsciously.

Medics may rely on *DSM-V* and its equivalents to make diagnosis and to determine suitable treatment for patients. At the moment scant medical attention is given to the principles of recovery as opposed to treatment. But maybe that is not as terrible as it may seem. Recovery is about the whole of a person's experience and relationships, so the medical element needs only to be one aspect – although the medics do need at least to be aware of what work is going on in other areas to support people in recovery and to make meaningful connections in support of their patients. And people seeking help need to be confident that the professionals helping them will respect and at least partly recognize their specific and individual experiences and circumstances.

One of my interviewees for this book – we'll call him David – was diagnosed and hospitalized as a young person with severe depressive episodes. He describes these periods as 'a shift in the nature of my day-to-day life. Empty. Hollow. Flat . . . I couldn't face going to work and I couldn't face telling my employer that I couldn't face going to work.' David was prescribed at various points different types of antidepressant, and later, lithium. He is not convinced that these prescriptions were always appropriate or properly 'indicated'. At one point a change in medication appeared to trigger a form of mania, and his problems got worse. David talks in most articulate terms about the difference between feeling understood and supported by the medical staff, and feeling that such understanding and support were lacking. 'The second psychiatrist had a lack of social skills. There was loads of pressure to take lithium. Sometimes the group CBT [cognitive behavioural therapy] seemed to expose vulnerabilities in some of the people.' He felt disempowered and in a sense forced to collude in his own disempowerment.

Later, when David was referred to a psychotherapist with whom he was able to establish a good and humorous rapport, 'I felt responded to rather than infantilized or feminized . . . I had jigsaw moments of self-awareness . . . Each time there were things I could build upon to help. The depressive episodes became less deep so I was able to make use of transformative moments in the therapy.'

David felt understood by this therapist and recognized *as himself*. He was able to bring to the therapeutic relationship an intelligent and sensitive critique of the medical conventions into which he had previously been expected to fit, and to contribute actively to his own recovery process: 'Reading and films were my self-medication. I stopped smoking weed [marijuana] and that definitely helped. The therapist pushed me a little bit too, and I appreciated that.'

David now works as a successful and respected clinical psychologist specializing in work with young people and families. He has a range of activities to help him stay well, including taking delight in time with his children, and makes use of his own experiences to provide an empathetic environment for his clients. 'I take pleasure in my ordinariness. I don't have to build a new Jerusalem. I don't take things for granted. I understand that depression is special, a kind of prison but also a safe space.' By safe space, perhaps what I understand David to be referring to is our fear of losing our sense of the familiar or our true self, an awareness of our inner fragility and a reluctance therefore to take direction or treatment from an external source (like a doctor) that does not recognize us *as we are*. We need to feel safe to move forward.

My late partner Chris mainly attempted to hide his condition, including from himself, and with some success. He refused to accept help for a long time, and when he did it was initially for anxiety and depression, not for addiction caused by lifelong and deep psychological anguish. Life and addiction became an excruciating balancing act. His need to deny, hide and deflect his awful behaviour and its consequences, and the help he had in doing so from his family, meant that as he became more ill he was ever more willing to cut across social norms. There was, and still is, a quadruple stigma for people like Chris to deal with before progress and recovery are possible: the stigma attached to not coping with adult responsibilities such as work and parenthood; the stigma attached to mental health problems of any kind; the stigma associated with facing up to one's past behaviour; and the specific and very toxic stigma attached to addiction itself, which of course is made stronger by the criminal nature of some types of substance misuse. It takes a good deal of bravery to face this, so when a person takes that step he or she needs safe space, recognition, encouragement and support – not condemnation. It is for good reason that a blog written by one of the participants in the RSA's recovery project was entitled 'Lions led by donkeys'.

Barriers to recovery

In the RSA's research into the lives of recovering heroin users,[11] people identified many barriers to recovery.

> Unsurprisingly, many of the factors that operated as barriers to recovery were the exact opposite of those which enabled recovery. For example, not being able to access treatment, not liking aspects of the treatment on offer, or feeling staff attitudes were negative or hostile could all dampen individuals' motivation to stay clean. Those in the study also often said that seeing other drug users was a real challenge to their recovery.
>
> 'Seeing people, you know. That's a challenge . . . All we've had is her [girlfriend's] family into our place . . . I'm not putting ourselves in risk like that, you know . . . because I just know the temptation . . . Even though I don't want to do it, I can't say if someone put it [heroin] in front of me what would happen. I'm not willing to risk that,' *Liam, aged 37*
>
> 'It's hard when you see someone . . . that look in their eyes and you can tell they're on something . . . kind of makes you jealous, you know . . . I want a feeling like that right now, kind of thing . . . It's hard to explain really. When you see someone really wasted you just think, "Wow, I wish I could feel that",' *Frances, aged 31*[12]

David, our interviewee, says that without the 'love, tolerance and support of my family I wouldn't be here', but for many of the RSA's interviewees family relationships are difficult:

Having stressful relationships with family members could equally be problematic, as was not having any friends who did not use [drugs].

My mum's attitude definitely [makes it difficult to stay clean]. Like I said, I can only talk for myself, but definitely for me it's my mum ... All I want my mum to do, I want my mum to sit and talk to me ... I've tried, but it ends up in an argument, so we just don't now. We find it easier not even to mention it [drug use]. *Beth, aged 31*

Addiction and the law

My focus in this book is on people's lived experiences, rather than on which side of a legal divide they may fall on, or any perceived moral argument: we will each take our own view about how to deal with questions of morality and legality. The practical point is that a recovery process has the potential to enable people to live well and sustainably in society, to take responsibility, to do as well as they can at a given moment, and to live peacefully with themselves and those around them. It should be noted that addiction and related mental health problems can trigger behaviour that sometimes crosses legal boundaries.

The *DSM-V* summary about the relationship (and confusion) between cultural considerations in different countries and law enforcement is very important. Much publicity has been given to the experience of the decriminalization of street drugs and progressive forms of support for addicts in Portugal, Switzerland and elsewhere. This book is not about to re-run those arguments, which have been made very well by health workers, campaigners and others, but it is useful even if obvious to note that where criminalization is a barrier to a person acknowledging a problem, or asking for help, then the consequences of that problem for the individual and for society are likely to continue unabated, with all that that entails.

Figures from the Prison Reform Trust give us pause for thought:

Approximately 200,000 children in England and Wales had a parent in prison at some point in 2009. This is more than double the number of children affected in the same year by divorce in the family. Fewer than 1% of all children in England are in care, but looked after children make up 30% of boys and 44% of girls in custody . . . 47% of children in custody in 2011–12 were there for non-violent crimes. 16% were there for a breach offence. 25% of children in the youth justice system have identified special educational needs, 46% are rated as underachieving at school and 29% have difficulties with literacy and numeracy. Of children interviewed in prison, 13% reported being regular crack users, and 11% had used heroin daily. In March 2011, 30% of children were held over 50 miles from their home, including 10% held over 100 miles away.[13]

Given what we understand about the strong correlation between addiction and crime, and between childhood trauma, family breakdown and later mental health problems including addictive behaviour, it looks from these statistics as if our prisons have somehow become factories for producing more addicts. An addiction therapist I met at the Priory Hospital said that for each addict there are on average a further nine people who are being adversely affected. That's a lot of damage.

Here are some more statistics from the Prison Reform Trust (reported from the end of December 2012). Of those prisoners who took drugs:

- 64 per cent reported using drugs in the four weeks before custody;
- 14 per cent of men and 15 per cent of women were serving sentences for drug offences;
- 55 per cent reported committing offences connected to their drug taking, with the need for money to buy drugs the most commonly cited factor;
- 48 per cent of women said they committed their offence to support someone else's drug use; the statistic for men was 22 per cent;
- among heroin users, on average women spent £50 per day on heroin compared to £30 for men;
- 19 per cent of those prisoners who admitted to using heroin reported first taking it in a prison.

Of those offenders who reported consuming alcohol in the previous year:

- 87 per cent of men and 75 per cent of women drank alcohol in the four weeks before custody;
- 32 per cent said they drank on a daily basis (daily drinking in the general UK population is around 16 per cent of men and 10 per cent of women) and drank an average of 20 units per day.[14]

In addition, in 44 per cent of violent crimes the victim believed that the offender was under the influence of alcohol. The Prison Reform Trust also found that men who returned to live with their partners were less likely to relapse and reoffend, while the opposite was true for women. Women prisoners were more likely to be in relationships with partners who abused drugs and committed crime, which tended to trigger relapse and reoffending.

What this tells us, if nothing else (as if we didn't know already), is that there is a strong relationship between offending and substance misuse, and that individual recovery solutions may vary by gender as well as for other reasons.

In the course of conversations leading to this book, I spoke with a probation officer who expressed considerable frustration about a new and, at that point, legal 'high' nicknamed 'spice', a synthetic cannabinoid that is intended to replicate the effects of cannabis. Prisoners were being routinely tested for cannabis, but because spice was a relatively novel substance there was as yet no standard test for it. Spice has been reported to have significant adverse effects. Yet prisoners were taking spice rather than cannabis, whose harms are felt to be fewer, because of the risk of punishment associated with being caught by testing. So regulation, which cannot keep pace with innovation in the manufacture of street drugs, was seen in the eyes of this probation officer to be actively contributing to harm rather than protecting either users or society.

This is an example of where an authoritarian, control- and treatment-led approach and the fixed *DSM-V* definition of substance use disorder or addictive disorder (the new edition includes gambling for the first time, as a behavioural illness separate from substance addiction) break down and lose their usefulness. By focusing on the substance and the syndrome rather than on people and their circumstances, the diagnosis and the proposed solution barely even address what is actually going on, and so have their own limitations and failure built in.

Recovery, not punishment

This is where the recovery movement has something much more powerful to say. Rather than negate and deny people's experiences, the idea of recovery is that people learn to live with the past and with their imperfections, and find positive steps forward that work for them:

> I always knew deep inside I would survive, albeit inside I felt and still do feel broken. Life throws things at you and you determine how you handle it and what it is going to do to you. I tried the alcohol, I tried the drugs, I tried all sorts of things to get rid of the feelings, to put them in a different place, to make them easier to cope with, but there is no other place – it is always there and it never goes away.
>
> Now I am older I don't want the feelings to go away. They are a big part of me – not the most important bit but important nonetheless – part of who I am and who I am becoming. Because of all my experiences I am learning to accept all of myself, feelings and all. Deep inside I always knew I would survive. I always had a determination to live a good and happy life and I believe I am succeeding.[15]

These are the words of 'June', who suffered years of abuse and unhappiness as a child, and finally found courage as an adult to take legal steps against her abuser. She had adopted a savvy, abrasive and streetwise personality to enable her to cope with feelings of intense pain and loss. Hard and brittle on the outside, she was in agony on the inside. For June's recovery, and against her earlier prejudices and expectations, she found that a counsellor helped:

> Counselling allowed me to be as honest as I could be at the time. I don't know if I ever got to the real depths of all my feelings or was one hundred per cent ready to look at myself that deeply but I do know that talking helped me immensely. It allowed me to find new ways of expressing myself, even my anger found a way to vent itself.

The kind of counselling support that June experienced was in the 'person-centred' tradition, which has philosophical links to what has become known as the recovery movement, and to related thinking about 'positive psychology' and 'social capital'. These jargon terms refer to ways of working and thinking that have produced real benefits for many people, so in the next chapter we will look at them to see what they might have to offer someone in mental distress.

The evidence that the medical view of treatment and recovery may be changing can be found in the official guidance provided to NHS staff by the National Institute for Health and Care Excellence.

For example, guideline 51, which was due for review in March 2015, is on alcohol-use disorders, and contains a specific section on person-centred care. A summary is given here:

- Treatment and care, and the information provided about it, should be culturally appropriate and take into account people's needs and preferences.
- Treatment and care, and associated information, should be accessible to people with additional needs such as physical, sensory or learning disabilities, and to people who do not speak or read English.
- Those receiving treatment should have the opportunity to make informed decisions about their care (unless they don't have the capacity to make such decisions or are under 16).
- Families and carers should have the opportunity to be involved in decisions about treatment and care, and be given the information and support they need in their own right.[16]

This sounds great, but of course doctors are busy people, with maybe only a ten-minute slot allocated for a first meeting with a patient. My observation of Chris's first such encounter with his GP was that he was able to deceive both the GP and himself as to the real nature of his difficulties, a trick he managed to pull off again and again in the context of the local mental health team and our hospital accident and emergency department (not to mention me). He was a long way from not feeling threatened or controlled, and the effect was that he threatened and controlled others. He rejected intervention and expressed something like contempt for the people offering it. A similar sentiment was expressed by an RSA workshop participant:

> When you go to Addaction or KCA and you try to explain these things you do get the impression that the person on the other side of the desk has only ever read it out of a book. And that is so patronising because they are saying you shouldn't feel like that, and you're like, hang on, you haven't got a clue.[17]

In another case in the same project, where for almost all of the participants their first port of call in seeking help was their GP, a participant said: 'When I first went to the doctors they were like, you're too young, you don't have an addiction. And I just kept getting turned away.' Where participants felt GPs got it right, this made a huge difference: 'The doctor's tone of voice changed – they were determined to get to the truth. And they did eventually.'

Sharing experience

According to research carried out by the charity Drugscope and an ICM poll, around one in five people have direct or indirect experience of drug addiction,[18] and according to the British Crime Survey almost 10 per cent of those between 16 and 59 used illegal drugs in 2009[19] – a figure rising to 20 per cent of those aged 16 to 24. The RSA's research suggests that the assets available to problem drug and alcohol users to help with their recovery, in the form of social networks, information resources, communications technologies and so on, are often overlooked. Informal social networks in particular seem to be important as they 'spread the contagious values and behaviours of well-being and hope that are integral to recovery'.[20]

Shared experience, in other words, and trust, and hope, are part of what is needed.

> I'm either going to get well or die. I didn't have any other choices. I was right at rock bottom. I had no housing. I was living on the streets, doing anything to get a drink.[21]

How do you go up from there?

3

Once in a lifetime: experiences of recovery and understanding 'what works'

Group facilitator: You came off it yourself?
Female workshop participant: Yeah, I found it took about three to four weeks. But I had Sam to help me a lot of the time.
Male workshop participant: I had just finished, just done my rattle, so I was quite supportive.
Female workshop participant: And I was just starting as he was coming out the other end of it, so I had him to help me through the main bit. He knew what I was going through and how I was feeling.[1]

For many people, the perception of having one's feelings and true self recognized and understood is essential to successful recovery. As the RSA report notes, a lot of people working in mental health and addiction services have experience of the problems they are helping with, either directly and personally (as with my interviewee David), or in those close to them, but for many reasons – sometimes as a matter of policy – they are unable to disclose that information to clients.

This can become a barrier to authentic communication, because withheld information can tip the balance of power in favour of the professional and cause anxiety or mistrust in the person needing help. Equally, however, too much disclosure from the professional can move the focus away from the person seeking help, and can tip vulnerable people away from expressing themselves honestly and getting in touch with the root of their problems – so it's a tricky balance that can only be managed with care, empathy and trust.

If your sense of your self is complex or uneasy, that too needs acknowledging:

I didn't recognize myself until I was in my 40s.

These are the words of Hilary, a transgender person who lived with a form of Asperger's syndrome and bipolar depression until well into middle age before being diagnosed and finding support and suitable ways to manage. Hilary's dissonant and jarring experience of 'self' contributed to long-term and serious mental health problems. He found being in groups especially difficult and needed long periods alone to recover from any group activity such as work, learning or socializing.

> Anxiety was my norm. Professionally I was in social work, but I got burnout, and I can't work now. In my mid-30s I was given SSRIs and tricyclics.[2] It was another transgender person who helped me recognize my symptoms and seek a diagnosis. With hindsight now I have much greater understanding of depression and I am seeking a peaceful place.

For Hilary, key components of ongoing recovery are:

- understanding your true self;
- understanding the nature of *your* particular challenges and what makes them difficult to handle;
- support and recognition from someone with comparable experience;
- access to the right kind of non-judgemental professional advice;
- anxiety management training;
- assertiveness training;
- the option to be alone when you want but able to connect with others when you feel like it;
- self-help books and art therapy;
- voluntary work helping others with similar problems.

For Hilary, photography also helps – a walk around town with a camera is a common way for him to de-stress after draining or anxiety-inducing experiences – and the support of peers was especially important, because 'I was not depressed enough to get an NHS care co-ordinator, but I was too complex for the system: I had to choose between my conditions, my gender question or my depression question, for which I attended art therapy. In the end the art therapist recommended me to a gender clinic . . . The diagnosis was a relief. The mask is off.'

Hilary's intelligent analysis of his dilemmas is notable: 'I tried to work but it was too much. Whether I was going to be able to cope was unpredictable. With volunteering I can contribute but opt out when I need to. Once you have a label though it can make you more sensitive to those aspects of your life, so it's important to keep balance. I don't have stamina but I find music helps.'

Gaps in services and potential for progress

On the basis of their detailed work with large numbers of people, the RSA report noted a number of gaps in provision, including:

> *Appointments with staff are too short and infrequent; inexperienced staff.*
> Most [participants in the research] agreed that the amount of time in meetings available to speak to care co-ordinators and/ or keyworkers was insufficient. An hour a week did not provide adequate opportunity to treat a person holistically and to meet their range of needs. It can take time to develop trusting relationships and to fully appreciate the underlying problems.[3]

Here are the other gaps noted in the report.

1 *Stigma and reintegration*: a lack of community engagement and understanding – although, as we saw in Chapter 2 from the Drugscope research, it may well be that the public is ahead of the policy-makers on this issue.
2 *Tension between experts by experience and experts by profession*: the many other imaginative recovery initiatives being tackled across the country (including this book) are all signs of progress with this longstanding problem.
3 *Lack of integration between services and advice*: the problem of 'joined-up thinking' that perennially affects public services. We can see real progress through the new local government responsibility for public health and other locally led primary care initiatives, such as the integration of medical and well-being support.[4]
4 *Dual diagnosis*: a lot of people have reported being passed from pillar to post and effectively having to choose which condition to have treated; when the problems are integrated the solution also needs to take into account all aspects of a person's experience. It was reported that some mental health professionals had a poor understanding of addiction and regarded problems associated with it as 'self-inflicted'.

5 *Friends and family*: involving friends and family in treatment can be complicated because they may be part of the problem, but many service users felt that under certain circumstances friends and family could be integral to recovery.

6 *Personalized treatment*: making people jump through a standard series of hoops does not produce very good results and as we have seen, can actually work against recovery. People need to develop a level of choice and control that works for them.

7 *Access and opening times*: the perpetual NHS and social services challenge. Often services are only available during office hours – fine if you aren't working, but what if you need help and have made sufficient progress to be able to work? And what about those tricky, dangerous times in the evenings and at the weekends when you are most likely to need support?

8 *Treatment services*: a lack of aftercare, a lack of meaningful activity, a lack of 'assertive outreach'.[5] This a primary gap that whole person recovery seeks to address, the ability of support to address the whole of a person's life and experience, rather than simply focusing on the 'problem'. Assertive outreach teams tend to be separate from conventional community mental health teams. Rethink, the mental health charity, describes it this way:

> They are specialist teams set up to work with you if you are an adult with a mental illness or personality disorder, and you find it difficult to work with services, have been admitted to hospital a number of times and may have other problems such as violence, self-harm, homelessness or substance abuse.
>
> Assertive Outreach Teams offer an intensive, long-term relationship with you to build up trust.
>
> These teams include staff with a mixture of skills to meet your needs.[6]

9 *Housing*: a propensity to either fail to help someone in housing need or to ghettoize people in recovery can compound people's problems. There is a balance to be found between enabling mutual support between people with common ground and trapping a person in an environment where recovery is prevented. Some participants have reported good experiences: one interviewee's encounter with Brighton Housing Trust was profoundly beneficial, and had involved not just supported

housing and empathetic staff but also skills training to enable him first to volunteer and then to re-enter paid work.

10 *Lack of hope*: a lot of experts by experience noted how important it is to 'feel and believe that things can improve'.[7] Focusing too much on the problem of 'rock bottom' or 'no light' can be counterproductive. It helps to hear other people's stories of hope and recovery.

Such gaps in provision can be deterrents and barriers to recovery. Research by the RSA and others shows that if these areas can be addressed, recovery is more likely to be successful.

Whole person recovery

As well as empathy, insight and recognition (support from others and understanding yourself), the RSA's Whole Person Recovery research mapped a series of factors that can contribute to well-being and successful recovery.

In Chapter 1 we began to consider the difference between treatment and recovery. The Mental Health Foundation defines recovery like this:

> In mental health, recovery does not always refer to the process of complete recovery from a mental health problem in the way that we may recover from a physical health problem.
>
> For many people, the concept of recovery is about staying in control of their life despite experiencing a mental health problem. Professionals in the mental health sector often refer to the 'recovery model' to describe this way of thinking.
>
> Putting recovery into action means focusing care on supporting recovery and building the resilience of people with mental health problems, not just on treating or managing their symptoms.
>
> There is no single definition of the concept of recovery for people with mental health problems, but the guiding principle is hope – the belief that it is possible for someone to regain a meaningful life, despite serious mental illness. Recovery is often referred to as a process, outlook, vision, conceptual framework or guiding principle.[8]

The RSA summarizes a person's recovery journey like this (as shown in Figure 1 on p. 14):

- *the baggage*: finding ways to manage past feelings and experiences;
- *breaking routines*: developing skills and capabilities for the future;
- *treatment*: formal and informal services and support;
- *making a plan*: formal and informal coping strategies;
- *the rest of my life*: getting well and staying well.

The first of these, baggage, can be a negative force, and may trigger relapse – but that need not be the end of recovery. *Relapse can be part of the recovery process*; it can lead to learning and greater insight, and may allow the person concerned to evolve new and different ways to cope. The other four elements on the list have a positive role in reinforcing each other – each works to make the next one stronger. In Chapters 4 and 5 I will explore in more detail things that people have tried to support their recovery.

So a key definition of 'recovery' is a process of *voluntarily sustaining progress towards health, well-being and productive and meaningful engagement in life and society*. This process might be supported and helped through a variety of means, but crucially its path, character and pace are shaped and determined by the individual whose journey it is.

Such a process has implications for the way that recovery services (as opposed to 'treatment' services) are designed:

> The objectives of 'recovery-oriented mental health services' are different from the objectives of traditional, 'treatment-and-cure' health services. The latter emphasizes symptom relief and relapse prevention. In recovery, symptomatic improvement is still important, and may well play a key role in a person's recovery, but quality of life, as judged by the individual, is central.[9]

There is now a great deal of research suggesting that this approach is more likely to be effective than old-fashioned non-consultative or coercive treatments.[10] Perhaps the most persuasive argument is personal testimony of the kind found in this book, but service users and service providers may differ in their understanding of what terms like 'consultative' or 'coercive' actually mean. Expectations on both sides need to be realistic, whether that relates to time-frames for treatment, budgets, tendency to relapse or the very availability of various types of service.

> Professionals tended to define successful treatment in terms of abstinence and harm reduction outcomes, while service users

tended to define 'success' in wider terms by identifying longer-term lifestyle goals such as being employed, securing housing, gaining education and skills, and improving family relationships.[11]

So as the National Treatment Agency (now part of Public Health England) makes tentative moves towards a greater focus on recovery, the empathetic and equal nature of communication between service user and service provider becomes ever more essential. For the simple reason that it won't work otherwise.

A note on abstinence and harm reduction

A lively public and professional debate has been raging for many years about the apparent conflict between 'harm reduction' and 'abstinence-based' approaches to treating addiction. Well-known author and comedian Russell Brand has led public discussion in recent times with his support for abstinence and his fearless reminders of the presence of substance misuse problems throughout society. Opposing views are articulated by many others.[12] This book will not advise anything except what works for you. The reason for this is that if, as seems often to be the case, a tendency to mental ill-health and/or addiction is rooted in early, serious or prolonged psychological suffering, then the recovery priorities must be psychological healing and an environment conducive to recovery, *supported* by treatment, not the other way around – and the nature of the healing process in a particular person will determine the nature of their treatment, if anything. The person comes first, not the system. As Hilary says:

> Now I can't separate the bipolar from the creative choice I have made to live the rest of my life. I'm lucky, I've had a lot of help. This is a beautiful city. I'm a visual person and there is always art and landscape.

The experiences of people who have had to learn the hard way how to manage their own treatment are salutary. Change is not easy and realism, self-care, kindness to oneself are intrinsic to the process:

> This month I'll probably stay at 25 [mg] because you don't want to come off it too quick. Because I have found in the past when I've come off it too quick I seem to go back on it . . . So at this stage I'll probably just stay, this month [and] probably just for

another month, just, you know, steady myself a bit more, and then [reduce]. *Annabel, aged 29*[13]

I think I'm in the right place and I'm doing alright. I hope I'm doing alright. It's gonna get harder before it gets easier. Um, I'm just waiting to sort of crack up a bit and that. But I think I'm doing alright, settling in and, um, I dunno, doing alright, I think. *Nathan, aged 30*[14]

My issue, work, I am finding a bit hard to do. But I am getting the help from my . . . peers . . . I've got to have two support groups twice a day, and I've got to talk about my feelings . . . But, yeah, it's really good. I'm getting a lot, I've been getting a lot done. *Stefan, aged 27*

To understand the need for recognition, self-care and kindness to yourself, it is helpful to look back at where these ideas come from and what triggered the research into their effectiveness in the first place.

A history of recovery

In 1934 an American alcoholic, Bill Wilson, became permanently sober, having spent several periods in hospital for treatment for his drinking. Experiencing sudden insight of a spiritual nature, he later founded what became Alcoholics Anonymous, a worldwide peer support group for recovering alcoholics with over two million members and around 100,000 separate groups in many different countries. AA is still a major, if not *the* major, form of peer support for recovering alcoholics, and participants may go along voluntarily themselves or may, as in the case of my late partner, be referred by medical staff. There are comparable support groups for affected families (Al-Anon) and for people affected by other drugs (Narcotics Anonymous). This peer support model is now widespread and is used for all manner of conditions and causes – I have even been involved in one for severe allergy. The key to the power of these groups and their effectiveness is the voluntary nature of participation and their capacity to allow people to share experiences.

Some people find the quasi-religious underpinning of AA's 'Twelve Step' programme off-putting; others find it helpful. The 'higher power' and prescriptive stages of the Twelve Steps are felt by some to provide essential structure for their ongoing recovery, as well as providing a space for them to work in the service of others.

For others, the sensation of coerciveness and not being true to one's own beliefs is a barrier. To find out more about the Twelve Step programme you can either get in touch with a local branch of AA (look online) or read *The Big Book*.[15] The main guide for people attending AA, this explains the steps and processes that it is felt members need to go through to achieve a life that is 'clean and serene'.

Freud and Jung

In the years before and beyond the foundation of AA in the first half of the twentieth century, Sigmund Freud and his pupil, colleague and later rival Carl Jung developed their psychological theories. Some of their ideas have been soundly debunked by later research, but their huge and fundamental achievement was to recognize, develop and legitimize the scientific study of the human mind. Many of us would find it hard now to imagine living without an idea of our 'unconscious' life, or describe ourselves without an understanding of how our childhood experiences formed us in some way. Of course writers and artists have always made the human mind part of their business. The difference with Freud and Jung was that they prepared the ground for the development of the academic field of psychology, so putting the study of the mind at the centre of both scholarly and public discussions about the nature of humanity. Freud also, by the by, helped legitimize and reintegrate sexuality and sexual expression as a normal part of human existence (even if again some of his ideas turned out to be a bit suspect). Critically, too, he established the idea that talking about inner worries and torment to an expert listener could alleviate psychological pain – the 'talking cure', or what we now call psychotherapy or counselling.

Jung expressed the idea of an inner life that had its own dynamism and motivations through the notion of the *anima* or *animus*, a kind of spirit, and he developed the theory of a 'collective unconscious' – a way of understanding connections and behaviours shared by people that are not subject to conscious control by the ego (the ego in this context, roughly speaking, is our conscious self). We could perhaps view co-dependency in this light.

In 1900 Freud published *The Interpretation of Dreams* (which was translated into English in 1953) and in 1901 *The Psychopathology of Everyday Life*. In the latter he makes clear that his theories apply to ordinary mental life, not only to 'pathological' states. Reading parts of *The Interpretation of Dreams* now, some sections stretch credulity, but anyone who has ever been afflicted by sleeplessness will recognize his urging of the importance to our mental well-being of the work done by our minds when we are asleep.[16]

Debate now focuses on whether the 'patient' or the therapist is the expert, and what exactly each is expert in – expert by profession or expert by experience? To see how the early theories developed to inform our present thinking about whole person or person-centred recovery, we need to look next at the work of an influential American psychologist, Carl Rogers.

Carl Rogers

Originally, Rogers worked in the mid-twentieth century with troubled children and he went on to lead the development of what has become known as 'person-centred' counselling. After looking at Freud and Jung, what strikes one about Rogers' work is both his humanity towards his clients and his utter focus on the person he is listening to, or counselling. Person-centred counselling differs in fundamental ways from, say, psychodynamic therapy, which is based on Freud's work and the idea of inner conflict, or cognitive behavioural therapy (CBT), which is often a fixed-term, learned, behavioural solution to a psychological problem. Many people speak well of their experiences of these two types of therapy, but in the context of a discussion about recovery they might be seen as tools in a toolkit: put simply, psychodynamic theory tends to assume the therapist is the 'expert' on the client's psychology, and CBT is a set of techniques for the localized management of distressing thoughts or behaviour rather than as a whole-person or whole-life approach, no doubt very effective for some but probably failing to address deep underlying causes of unhappiness. Research on the benefits of different types of therapy suggests, revealingly, that the determining factor in the success or failure of psychotherapy is the *quality of the relationship* between client and counsellor.

Sceptics look at Rogers' radically non-directive approach to counselling and question how it can possibly be beneficial for people in mental distress, offering as it does no bespoke solutions, no twelve steps, no 'treatment', literally no direction. It is helpful therefore to look at the ideas that underpin person-centred practice, much of it supported by research, to see why it has become globally recognized as a form of psychotherapy.[17]

Many people will be familiar with the notion that psychological harm in childhood can cause mental health problems in adult life. In helping clients to develop insight into their own difficulties, Rogers focuses on what he calls 'conditions of worth'. Essentially, these are the conditions under and upon which we develop a sense of being loved and valued as children. So if, as we grow up, we receive love unconditionally in a perfect and flawlessly caring and stimulating environment (and who gets that?), then we will in theory develop as our true selves, able to feel and express the range of human emotions freely and healthily.

No one does get that, of course, and for many or most people feeling loved and valued in our childhood was contingent at least some of the time on certain behaviours or responses: being 'good', being quiet, not crying, being 'brave', not challenging authority of whatever kind, passively accepting the way things are, keeping out of the way, not 'telling' and so on. For some people the consequences of not abiding by these codes can be very damaging indeed, and may involve the withholding of love, emotional neglect, physical 'punishment', psychological abuse and more. As a way to present the 'correct' and desired behaviour being asked of us we can develop a false version of ourselves for coping and self-preservation purposes. The result of this is inner conflict between the self we feel ourselves to be and the self we feel the world expects of us. Conditions of worth can be created by parents, grandparents, siblings and carers, of course, but also by teachers, partners and other figures of influence and authority in our lives. We 'repress' or hide our emotions (even from ourselves) in order to survive and win (or try to win) their approval. Supporting people to get back in touch with themselves, in the world, as they are, and to become whole rather than fragmented or conflicted is at the heart of what person-centred care is about.

How difficult it can be for a person to deal with returning emotions at the beginning of the recovery journey is revealed by participants in the RSA work:

> I don't know, I just found it so intense . . . I had all these feelings starting to come that I didn't like feeling, you know . . . I felt incredibly agitated. Incredibly uncomfortable. *Debbie, aged 28*

Before I had no emotions. I was too interested in getting high. *Isabelle, aged 35*

I never used to cry at all. In fact, I'd do my damnedest to stop myself crying. Because it's not a man thing, is it . . . ? But yeah, I did cry a couple of times in rehab . . . Nothing would have touched me that deeply before. *Nathan, aged 30*[18]

Carl Rogers argued that for beneficial therapeutic change to occur in a person, some basic or 'core' conditions need to exist in the relationship between counsellor and client: empathy, 'unconditional positive regard' and 'congruence'.

In order to be empathetic, the counsellor needs to be able to 'feel with' and 'walk alongside' you, without making assumptions (at all) and without seeking to impose his or her own interpretation of your experiences of emotions. That includes not asking leading questions or seeking to impose any order or direction on the conversation that is not welcome to the client. The counsellor must be a highly expert and experienced listener to be at all effective. Anyone who has tried to learn listening skills formally will testify how difficult that is to accomplish. No interrupting, no value judgements, no 'over-sharing' or 'me too'. But critically, as well as *feeling* empathy, the counsellor must be able to *express* empathy in a way that the client trusts, in order for that client to feel he or she is in a safe and non-judgemental space. This means person-centred counsellors use a lot of nodding and non-verbal cues to let someone know that they are being heard and understood. If you are accustomed to behaving according to your conditions of worth, and this has caused you mental anguish, you are not going to let your barriers down to a complete stranger without being pretty sure they 'get' you. This is (obviously) particularly important in the context of recovery dialogues that cross cultural, gender, race, class or religious or other boundaries, and where existing mental health treatment services may have come up against problems in the past:

They don't want to come forward because they're scared . . . There's no Asian there . . . there's no-one working there that they can talk to. OK, you can get a translator but I wouldn't be comfortable, you know if my wife came there she wouldn't be comfortable with a man translating . . . [Having Asian people in the services] would

help a lot. Do you know why? Because they'll come forward. At
the moment they're suffering. Loads of families.[19]

To give a further example of why trust and empathy are so
important: when I was facilitating a workshop for women in
recovery, the participants were generous enough to share many
personal stories. They talked about their fear of seeking help from
'official' sources because they knew other women whose children
had been taken into care. For some this meant their problems
simply got worse, and in more than one case they ended up in the
hands of the criminal justice system as a result of their problems
and lost their children to state care anyway.

One woman's experience particularly sticks in the memory. She
got up courage to seek help and was referred to residential rehab.
Her mental distress originated in sexual abuse. At rehab she was
asked to participate in group therapy to talk about her difficulties –
where all of the other participants were men. The inappropriateness
of this is shocking (and the fact that such women go through it
truly amazing) – but critically, from the point of view of whole
person recovery and person-centred support, there appears in this
scenario a complete absence of empathy.

Rogers' next core condition, 'unconditional positive regard', is
a fancy way of saying you value someone positively and without
any prejudice: you can show warmth and acceptance for that
person as a human being regardless of his or her identity or experience. Imagine safe companionship, complete acceptance. 'It is an
attitude of the counsellor . . . This attitude of acceptance towards
the client is not only consistent from client to client but endures
throughout the person-centred counsellor's relationship with any
one client.'[20] It is not just being 'nice', but offering genuine warmth
and kindness.

So as a client seeking, in this example, counselling help with your
recovery, you can have confidence that the counsellor empathizes
with you without judgement, and feels warm and accepting towards
you. Do you trust the counsellor yet? For us to trust anyone, we
need to feel that that person respects us enough to be himself or
herself in our presence. This is where Rogers' third core condition,
'congruence', comes in. If our recovery depends on us being in a
safe and empathetic environment long enough to explore what is

fundamentally troubling us and to work out how to move towards being more well in ourselves – and that meanwhile risks making ourselves open and vulnerable – then it is critical that the person we are allowing to facilitate that safe environment knows how to be himself or herself, so that we can get the measure of that person and understand the nature of the environment he or she creates. We need to trust the person, in other words. Congruence is knowing how to be one's authentic self, and being self-aware enough to live with and manage that self, including one's emotions and reactions. It is a key skill for person-centred counsellors.

> It took me ages to 'get it' as far as congruence was concerned. I was brought up as a nice British girl who was always careful to be polite and never to say bad things to people . . . I had been brought up to fear my congruence was dangerous. It might be my incongruence that was damaging.[21]

So as a resource for whole person recovery, you can see how the philosophy of person-centred counselling is a vital ingredient, even if a person doesn't actually seek counselling. At the heart of the process is self-acceptance, safe space, trust, learning, human warmth and kindness.

If we remind ourselves of the key components of whole person recovery, we can see that the person-centred philosophy (i.e. putting the person first, not the system or idea) reinforces each stage of recovery:

- *the baggage*: finding ways to manage past feelings and experiences;
- *breaking routines*: developing skills and capabilities for the future;
- *treatment*: formal and informal services and support;
- *making a plan*: formal and informal coping strategies;
- *the rest of my life*: getting well and staying well.

Isolation

> It's a multitude of what you've learnt along the way and your acceptance of what you've learnt. Otherwise you would still be out there.[22]

Out there. One of the most painful and hard-to-manage aspects of any mental health disorder for the person concerned is increasing social isolation and loneliness: difficulties ranging from dealing with money and work to maintaining relationships and a home, even trouble getting up in the morning or going to sleep at night, can all put unbearable strain on our coping mechanisms and social/family connections. Given what we already know about many underlying causes of mental suffering, and the conditions needed to create sustainable recovery, why do we (by which I mean decision-makers as well as everybody else) expect people to cope on their own so much of the time? For some people, as I have already said, family or social networks can be part of the problem, but for others they are literally lifesavers.

> If it wasn't for my mum I would be dead by now.

> I turn to my friends and family. The Macmillan nurse team. My community psychiatric nurse. My keyworker at the housing trust.[23]

Disgraced journalist, contrite plagiarist and former addict Johann Hari puts it succinctly:

> What I learned is that the opposite of addiction is not sobriety. The opposite of addiction is human connection.[24]

Human connection can only be (re)built in the context of trust. Hari would earn approval from many in AA for his recognition of past bad behaviour and addictive thinking:

> Look . . . I can talk to you about why what happened in my life happened. But I just think that's a way of trying to invite sympathy, and that would be weaselly. If you tell a detailed personal story about yourself, you're inherently asking people to sympathise with you, and actually I don't think people should be sympathetic to me. I am ashamed of what I did. I did some things that were really nasty and cruel.

He almost has a winning point. Yet, speaking from the point of view of someone who was on the receiving end of 'weaselly' and 'nasty and cruel' behaviour perpetrated by an addict, I maintain critical distance when I wonder if someone may be competing now not to be the most grand or important or talented but the best at self-hatred. Acceptance of one's own ordinariness and regular human dimensions seems to be a key resource in recovery from the affliction of addiction.

The person that convinced me of this, other than Chris in his brief flirtation with recovery, is author Abraham Twerski. His description of addictive thinking not only helped me get to grips with what had been going on in my relationship, but also – rather unexpectedly – helped me understand my own addiction to cigarettes, and despite the traumatic events that I was going through at the time motivated me to give up smoking after almost 30 years as a smoker. I was able to bypass my addiction and reconnect with my primary relationships with my daughter, my own health and, quite frankly, common sense.

Putting together what you need to sustain this process of re-linking a person to the world and others around him or her in healthy and sustainable ways is called building 'recovery capital', and we will look at this in Chapter 4. A range of other resources, varying from place to place and person to person, can be called upon, and some of these are listed at the end of the book.

Addiction in social context

Seeing personal pain in its social context, and understanding how addiction in particular and the mental health crisis in general might be products of the way we live and the way we organize society, has been the subject of eye-catching research by the Canadian psychologist Bruce Alexander. His book *The Globalization of Addiction: A study in poverty of the spirit* was published by Oxford University Press in 2008. He argues that Western society has tried 'all the religious, coercive, medical and compassionate solutions' and that we will only be able to attend properly to the full extent of the problem when we recognize its social and economic causes. He gave a talk at the RSA entitled 'Addiction: what to do when all else has failed',[25] and he summarizes his view as follows:

> History shows that addiction can be rare in a society for many centuries, but can become nearly universal when circumstances change – for example, when a cohesive tribal culture is crushed or an advanced civilization collapses. Of course, this historical perspective does not deny that differences in vulnerability are built into each individual's genes, individual experience, and personal character, but it removes individual differences from the foreground of attention, because societal determinants are so much more powerful. Addiction is much more a social problem than an individual disorder.[26]

In particular Alexander documents how dramatic economic or social change, forced migration and other products of globalization are associated with similarly dramatic increases in addiction and related mental health problems. Whether you think 'all else has failed' or rather that we need to change strategy or work harder towards person-centred approaches, my own feeling is that it is helpful for people who have the time, energy and inclination to look at some of Bruce Alexander's ideas, not least because they have the potential to dilute the force of shame, blame and stigma that is such a toxic barrier to recovery.

> The conventional wisdom depicts addiction, most fundamentally, as an individual problem. Some individuals become addicted and others do not. An individual who becomes addicted must somehow be restored to normalcy. There is an odd dualism built in to this individual-centred depiction: addiction is seen either as an illness or as a moral defect or – somehow – both at once.[27]

The point here is that, to quote the poet, 'no man is an island' and that where the roots of mental ill-health lie in previous suffering, as is often the case with addiction and other conditions such as anxiety and depression, then this is indeed a social as well as an individual phenomenon. Whole person recovery therefore means the recovery of a person in society, the recovery of healthy relationships, not merely the recovery of a private individual who could otherwise be chastised and blamed.

4

It's not yesterday any more: creating recovery – a personalized path to a better life

So maybe you, or a person you care for, has reached the point of recognizing there is a problem and that change is needed. Possibly you feel confident. Possibly you are terrified. Both are good. Maybe you have also recognized the stresses, events, people and activities that can trigger relapse, and thought about ways you can move away from those and be less affected by them. Perhaps by this stage you are resolving to take action, or have already done so. If you are exceptionally brave, you may have taken on board that you probably cannot do this on your own (and that applies to experts by profession as well as experts by experience). Building your 'recovery capital' will help you on your journey, even if you falter or make mistakes. People have been there before and you are not alone.

> 'No matter what happens, you don't have to pick up a drink or drug today.' These words tend to strike fear in the hearts of many alcoholics and addicts who are new to recovery.

Georgia W. shares her suggestions and advice in *Don't Let the Bastards Grind You Down*, from which these words are taken.[1] A funny and frank writer, she is full of insights – from how to hold on to your honesty and integrity, to how to have sober sex. Her focus is on the early stages of recovery, and how to avoid common pitfalls. On relapse she says:

> Someone once told me that I'd never have to drink or drug again, once I'd decided to quit. It didn't take me long to come up with a mental response: 'Wow, really? Why don't you take that golden nugget of wisdom and shove it up your ass?' . . . A recovery program gives us tools to use, which we need to use before we get to the point where the tiger is stirring and the disease is awake. Having a system in place allows us to recognize the negative feel-

ings and protect ourselves by becoming mentally and spiritually fit. That way, when we let our guard down, there are backups in place. There are friends we can call, recovery meetings we can go to, or even books we can read.[2]

This chapter, then, is about creating your personalized recovery 'system' or 'capital', mapping the resources you need to go forward, to tap into your inner instinct and tendency to get well and stay well. By 'resources', I mean anything that you can call upon for help, comfort, information, enjoyment and support: friends and family (but only if they are helpful); professionals such as doctors, counsellors, community workers, advice workers; tutors, courses and other sources of learning; creativity, writing, sport or other leisure activities; trusted prescribed medication or various forms of therapy, if that is part of what benefits you; massage, aromatherapy, meditation, mindfulness, if those help; work, training, volunteering or other types of occupation; peer support and listening; and yes, of course, money.

Georgia W. recommends recording and celebrating the 'firsts' of your recovery journey, your personal milestones and achievements: your first sober birthday; your first successful volunteering day; your first date; even your first break-up. Marking and remembering the newness and specialness of these achievements is important. Don't be embarrassed to congratulate yourself.

> One of the best ways to combat the feelings of alienation we often experience at family or social events is to take along a sober friend. Having someone in the 'trenches' with you is one of the most responsible actions you can do to safeguard your recovery and your state of mind . . . Recognize a birthday or anniversary for what it is: a chance to reflect on the previous year and see how far you've come. In time, you will actually start enjoying those milestones instead of suffering through them.[3]

There are any number of ways you can 'map' or find out about the recovery resources ('capital') available to you. The NHS and the charity sector offer a wide range of information, advice and support. You will also have informal and unofficial forms of support that may be just as powerful as these, or more so. And it really helps to do this with other people, because the more minds and networks you can access for the benefit of your recovery, the more choices and back-up you have. Two examples of ways to do this are 'asset mapping' and EXACT groups. Other tools, including the 'recovery star', are covered in the next chapter.

Asset mapping

In the early 1980s, riots broke out in a number of British cities. In Brixton in south London, there was effectively an uprising in protest at racism, poor social and economic conditions, and a history of brutal policing, especially the 'sus' laws, which saw many young black men in particular stopped and searched on the street for drugs and weapons. Many politicians were perplexed: there had been numerous policy interventions and initiatives aimed at 'solving' problems in the borough, but still people were rioting. How could that be?

As a result of these events, Lord Scarman, QC was charged with setting up an inquiry into their causes and potential solutions. What emerged was the profound disempowerment of local people, who had barely been consulted about the great initiatives put forward by policy-makers in response to the area's social problems, let alone had any proper say in or democratic control over what happened. What was needed was a way of genuinely shifting power and decision-making to make use of what the local people knew and saw, and to allow them to determine for themselves the local priorities for action, and what might be the Brixton community's preferred solutions. The process of working on an equal basis with groups of people and whole communities to design and deliver plans and projects has become known as 'asset-based community development' (ABCD),[4] and the same principles are now being extended and combined with 'person-centred' thinking to build 'recovery communities'.

To understand the process of shifting from top-down direction to localized control (which you might even call *democracy* or, in its theoretical sense of 'no government', *anarchy*), and how that might help recovery, it is useful to look at the 'ladder of participation' (see Figure 2 on p. 46) developed by Sherry Arnstein and published in, of all places, the *Journal of the American Institute of Planners* in 1969.[5] Bear with me!

Many people struggling with mental health problems and/or addiction will recognize their position in relation to services to

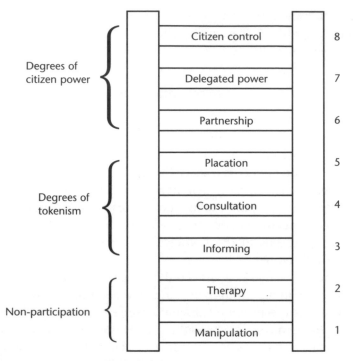

Figure 2 The ladder of participation

be somewhere between 1 and 3 on the ladder. Stages 3 to 5 can be understood perhaps to be the kind of position that so enrages people who are struggling and that alienates them from receiving *real help that actually works*. Stages 6 to 8 might describe the process by which the people of Brixton implemented serious and beneficial changes for their community that boosted jobs, businesses and local services, as well as reducing violence.

A similar process can be applied in building recovery capital and recovery communities. With experts by experience and experts by profession working *together*, many otherwise hidden resources, connections, networks, ideas and activities can be unlocked for the benefit of people in recovery and, by reducing the incidence and cost of problems associated with, for example, drug misuse, for the benefit of wider society and the public purse. *Our money gets used for us*, in other words, rather than for projects and services that keep a small number of disconnected professionals in business, and services are designed with, around and for the people who use them.

We should not underestimate people's capabilities and common sense. For example, in West Sussex a recovery partnership was established as a result of the RSA study and other research. Service users were asked whether they wanted to exercise control over budgets. A small majority were against, as they did not at that stage feel confident enough to do so effectively. But the real possibility was there and people chose what suited them at that stage of the project and at that stage of their involvement and recovery.

At a workshop at the Brighton Festival Fringe in 2014, I asked participants to do an exercise to map the 'assets' we had in the room. We spread out huge pieces of paper on the floor, with different headings for the kinds of things we were trying to identify. The theme of the workshop was recovery, reading and well-being. Each participant had some coloured sticky notes, and then was asked to jot down his or her thoughts and place them under each heading, as ideas occurred. Some people did this silently, while for others it was beneficial to chat and exchange thoughts. In the end we had something that looked like the collection of boxes in Figure 3 (pp. 48–9).

This enormous and varied collection of skills, enthusiasms, connections, ideas, knowledge and abilities was put together by seven people who barely knew each other, without preparation, in 15 minutes. A majority were not in paid employment. It is worth noting how often there appear links that would not have emerged had we formally focused only on people's professional identity or skills. For example, the person who was looking to get more local people involved in exercise might not have known to make a connection with either the tennis coach or the former triathlon runner because their current or former paid work fell into an entirely different domain, so any communication via formal professional and organizational networks would have missed a fantastic local asset.

This, as well as the problems associated with the power being in the wrong place, is why assuming that the professionals on their own can solve society's challenges (including mental health challenges and our personal suffering) is doomed to failure. Questions at the workshop about formal sources of support such as college and grant-awarding bodies got far fewer responses than some of the other questions, but the exercise brought our two or three people with fundraising skills and an awful lot more with the ability to

Work I do
Work in hostels
Mental health care
Book promotion
Keyworker
Fundraising
Reception/admin
Dental nursing

Professional advice I use
State benefits
Debt advice
Housing
Doctor
Personal advocacy

Languages I can speak
English
French
Spanish
German
My own language that no one else knows yet

Volunteering I do
Recovery/rehab
Community allotment/gardening
Allergy support group
Recycling
Art workshops
I am a book in a human library
I am a recovery sponsor
Blog about well-being

Organizations I have links to
Royal Institute of British Architects
Macmillan Cancer Care
The National Health Service
The Royal Society of Arts
Narcotics Anonymous
Brighton Housing Trust
Cambridge University
A local charity for people with Asperger's syndrome and high functioning autism
A local charity offering support for transgender people
The General Dental Council
Mind, the mental health charity
Mind Out, the mental health charity for lesbian, gay, bisexual and transgender people
The City Council

Things I enjoy
Talking with people
Playing music
Smiling
Watching films
Eating
Reading
Art
Writing
Photography
Walking
Being with friends
Learning new skills
Laughing
Listening to loud music
Books
Theatre
Travelling
Cross-stitch
Chocolate
Sitting in the sun
Reading to children
Country walks every Thursday
A really hot bubble bath and a book

Courses I have done
Architecture
Art psychotherapy
Counselling skills
Horticulture
Child protection
Teaching adult basic skills
Teaching creativity
Working with vulnerable adults
Advocacy
Colour therapy
Dental nursing and oral health
English literature
Project management
Budgeting

Skills I have
Patience
Organization
Graphic design
Writing
Proofreading and editing
Art
Listening
Nursing
Project management
Photography
Teaching
Mediation

Places I go
India
Trinidad
Bed. Zzzzz
Churches
The library
To the sea
Theatre
Cinema
The Isle of Wight
The park
London
National Trust places
Outside

Things I want to learn
Italian
Patience
To sing in front of people
To like myself
Spanish
Singing
To keep my opinions to myself
How to be happy
Piano
How to love openly
Hula hooping
Guitar
British Sign Language
Architecture
More photography skills

Clubs and societies I belong to
British Wheel of Yoga
Alcoholics Anonymous
The local running club
A small business IT support club
An allergy support group
The National Trust
Assert
The Royal Society of Arts

A local problem I would like to tackle
Mental health/depression
Street drinking
Homelessness
Drug and alcohol misuse
Traffic jams
Dog poo on the pavements
Child literacy
Greed
Getting people to do more exercise
World peace
Inequality

Things I can teach
Budgeting
Yoga
Customer care
Information retrieval systems

Things I am really good at
Jumping
Understanding other people's perspective
Dancing
Colour – artistic creation and décor
Communicating verbally with others
Listening
Art
Playing samba shakers
Patience
Moaning

People I love
My family
My son and cats
Parents, husband, children
My daughter Maria
Too many to list
My family and the dog

People I turn to for help
Counsellor
Bodyworker
Advocate
Sponsor
Friends (twice)
Siblings
My great friend
Doctor
The Macmillan team
Friends and family
My sponsor
The housing trust worker
Siblings

People I Know that give out grants
NHS
The National Lottery

Things I am responsible for
Too much
My own well-being
Child, cats, myself
Cat
Me
Community Links Service
Dog (twice)

The kind of person I am
A 'try hard' person
Generous
A bit OCD (obsessive compulsive disorder)
Silly
Sensitive
Fragile
Determined
Disgusting
Open
Scared
Capable
Sociable
Smiley
Multi-faceted

Things I do for my health
Walk
Yoga
Dance
Eat very healthy food
Go to a reading group
Walk my dog
Eat fruit

Things that make me feel hopeful
People being kind
When someone says 'thank you'
People who care about the planet
Attending self-help groups
Encouragement from a friend
People, friends

Problems I have solved
My own housing
Many, but very few on my own
How to move and not move
My own mental health

People who love me
Parents, daughter, friends
Mum/dad
My son and dad
Everyone that I love
Husband, children, close family, friends

Things I do to cheer myself up
Phone a friend
Eat lots of cake
Reading
Chat with a friend
See friends for coffee or drinks
Eat curry or chocolate
Watch a comedy
Cuddle my husband
Listen to music
Sit in the sunshine

My skills
Speak German
Coach tennis
Laughing at my own jokes
Talking through other people's problems
Good listener
Dancing
Talking with all sorts of people
Organizing

I know about . . .
Books
Photography
Cooking
Dementia
Triathlon
Motor racing
Tennis
Gardening

My college
Open University
Sussex Downs College of Further Education
Cambridge University

My work
Volunteering
Library online resources
Frustrated
I hate getting up for work

Links to medical support
NHS
Visit GP
Care worker
Nursing

Links to charity
People Can/Scarman Trust
Macmillan Cancer Care
Animal rescue
Fundraising
Caring
Community action trust

Links to friends
Supportive
Fun memories
Local
Priceless
Teresa – she is always there for me
Everyone is a potential friend
Wonderful
Lovely friends that I cherish and love

Links to colleagues
They support my work
Team
Enthusiastic and committed
My jobshare partner makes me look again at what I do

Figure 3 Recovery assets

share their skills and knowledge with others. Money and learning are both vital components of recovery capital but they may not be where you think they are, as the above process shows.

It is also worth noting that asking similar questions with different emphasis – 'Things I can teach' and 'Courses I have done', for example – got very different answers, so it's important to keep an open mind and be willing to make imaginative leaps.

So to develop your own recovery capital you might take a similar approach, collaborating with people you trust and who can help you, at a pace that suits you.

EXACT groups

One of the ways people have put together recovery capital is by creating self-run peer support networks, sometimes known as EXACT groups – groups of ex-addicts who collaborate and provide mutual support.

In West Sussex, EXACT groups were set up in both Crawley and Bognor Regis. As well as providing the shared safe space, dialogue, understanding and kindness that people needed, these groups participated in the local 'Recovery Partnership' on a (more or less) equal footing with professionals in the drug and alcohol action team and other key organizations, such as homelessness charities, the police, housing associations and the NHS. Along the way, EXACT group members became highly skilled in consultation and representation skills. They were able to provide advice and guidance to the partnership, and they led the development of new projects, such as a 24-hour online recovery-focused radio service and the Small Sparks scheme, a community grants programme offering modest sums to recovering users to allow them to take the next step on their recovery journey. Recovery may fail due to a relatively small obstacle, such as having insufficient funds for transport to a job interview, or to re-engage socially by, for example, joining the local leisure centre. The Small Sparks scheme carried minimal risk to the service providers (the greater risk was to the service user) and was conspicuously successful.

5

Other recovery tools

The recovery star

The 'recovery star' is a tried and tested tool for people managing their recovery, developed by an organization called Triangle along with the Mental Health Providers Forum. Much of the material is copyright, and training and a licence are required to adopt the techniques in professional settings. Anyone, however, can preview the material by subscribing to the mailing list at <www.outcomesstar. org.uk/signup/>. There are adapted versions for mental health, alcohol misuse, ADHD, domestic abuse and a range of other circumstances.

The recovery star has ten 'points' covering ten areas of life, with a 'ladder of change' on which we can map our progress. The star is a visual representation of where we are in our recovery. It helps keep the inevitable complexity of life under control and makes it easier to understand by creating a simple diagram. This is how the star is explained:

> At one end of a point on the star is the feeling of being *stuck* – of not feeling able to face the problem or accept help.
>
> From stuck we move to *accepting help*. At this stage we want to get away from the problem and we hope that someone else can sort it out for us.
>
> Then we start *believing* – that we can make a difference ourselves in our life. We look ahead to what we want as well as away from what we don't want. We start to do things ourselves to achieve our goal as well as accepting help from others.
>
> The next step is *learning* how to make our recovery a reality. It's a trial and error process. Some things we do work, and some things don't, so we need support through this process.
>
> As we learn, we gradually become more self-reliant until we can manage without help from a project.[1]

From Bruce Alexander's (see p. 41) point of view, the recovery star may be seen as overly focused on the individual and insufficiently focused on society's role. Nonetheless, many people have found this way of analysing their circumstances very helpful.

The ten areas of life that the star looks at are:

- managing mental health
- physical health and self-care
- living skills
- social networks
- work
- relationships
- addictive behaviour
- responsibilities
- identity and self-esteem
- trust and hope.

People can look at where they are on the scale from 'stuck' to 'self-reliant' in each of these areas, either alone or ideally working with someone they trust, such as a key worker, and can seek appropriate information, advice and guidance about the next steps. For example, with regard to trust and hope, which are central to our concerns with recovery in this book, this is about having

> a sense that there are people you can trust and there is hope for your future. It is about trusting in others, trusting in yourself and ultimately having faith in life and trusting that things will work out somehow. It might help to ask yourself who you trust when things get very tough? And do you have faith that, whatever happens, you or someone out there will find a way through?[2]

NHS self-assessment

A much quicker and less thorough version of this process is commonly used for mental health assessments by the NHS, using GAD-7 and PHQ-9 scores. What it lacks in comprehensiveness the assessment makes up for in speed and focus – both undoubtedly essential in a system where psychological maladies are so embarrassingly under-addressed and under-budgeted compared with physical illnesses. GAD stands for 'generalized anxiety disorder' and the scoring sheet is used for simple self-assessment. The professionals use the results as a screening tool and to try to establish the severity of a person's suffering.

GAD scoring is based on rigorous research, but of course as a self-assessment tool it is only as useful as the accuracy of the responses, which are determined by our degree of self-knowledge and how readily we are prepared to share our insight with professionals and record it. The nature of our individual personalities mean we may answer questions in different ways and underplay or overplay specific symptoms or feelings. For identifying generalized anxiety, the GAD process is seen to be 80 to 90 per cent accurate. For other forms of anxiety, such as panic disorder and social anxiety, it is seen as slightly less effective but still moderately accurate, and for post-traumatic stress as useful but less effective. You can do the test here: <www.patient.co.uk/doctor/generalised-anxiety-disorder-assessment-gad-7>.

It is an exercise that you can repeat from time to time if you find it helpful to track certain aspects of progress on your recovery, such as how well you are able to relax or how quickly you become irritable.

PHQ-9 is a comparable assessment questionnaire that looks at the relative severity of depression and how well someone is responding to treatment. The NHS primary care trust in the area where I live uses GAD-7 and PHQ-9 together. PHQ-9 can also be used by professionals to make a tentative diagnosis with people in at-risk groups. A preliminary assessment can be done using the PHQ-2 questionnaire developed in parallel. You can do the PHQ-9 test here: <www.patient.co.uk/doctor/patient-health-questionnaire-phq-9>.

If you are concerned by your scores you should, naturally, seek support, perhaps from a GP, a telephone helpline or your local mental health service. Very often, if your difficulties include the use of alcohol, street drugs, prescription drugs or addictive behaviour like compulsive gambling, you can refer yourself directly to your local drug and alcohol service without having to go through your doctor, although referral through a GP is still a common route. Search online for 'mental health team' or 'drug and alcohol action team', or contact your local branch of a mental health charity such as Mind or Addaction, who will be able to point you in the right direction.

None of these processes is perfect, of course, and they are most likely to work better if you are self-aware and feel active in your own recovery. Chris, my late partner, was initially diagnosed with anxiety and depression. When I first met him he told me he was prone to panic attacks. At one point he certainly succumbed to psychosis. He had difficulties with managing anger and resentment. He was fundamentally co-dependent in his family relationships. He was profoundly affected by all of those things, but it was only after a somewhat challenging few days (for him) of engagement with a residential rehab environment that he felt safe enough to even *start* engaging with the more intractable problem of his addictions. I wish I had known then what I know now about how much support, experience and kindness was available locally to help us, including from the NHS – even though the NHS entirely failed to spot the character of Chris's problems on its first, second and third opportunities.

The charitable and voluntary sector

As well as a number of important national charities working to ameliorate a variety of mental health conditions including addiction, there are lots of local or specialist charities and support groups dealing with, for example, housing, campaigning and family support. Examples of these are included in the 'Helpful organizations' section; it would be impossible to list them all. Given the importance of local knowledge, networks and support to recovery, a great asset will be to talk to people who are going through recovery already and ask for recommendations. In my home city, there is a community hub and a Council for Voluntary Services that are invaluable sources of information. Even after the devastating budget cuts of the post-2008 austerity measures, these organizations can give access to valuable peer support and expertise. They exist in most parts of the UK and if you want to find charities, voluntary groups and people who share your experiences they are a good place to start. You can search online or contact your local authority for contact details, or alternatively contact either the Citizens' Advice Bureau (if you can get through – their services are massively in demand) or the National Council for Voluntary Services, <www.ncvo.org.uk>, who should be able to give you information about organizations in your area that deal with your condition or questions.

In rural areas it can be trickier, for a number of reasons, to find support. First of all, the problem of stigma in the 'village goldfish bowl' where everyone knows each other's business can be a powerful barrier to seeking help. Second, the dispersed nature and lower density of the population means it is often not cost-efficient to provide services in these areas. Third, getting to the places where services *are* provided can be difficult in the absence of effective public transport.

Generally, the reported incidence of mental health problems and addiction is slightly lower in rural areas than in urban ones; that may be due to a combination of relatively stable and well-networked communities on the one hand, or to greater social isolation and lower reporting of the problems that do actually exist on the other. To find out what is available, an online search may help (if you can get decent broadband in your area), or you could try your local 'rural community council'. These organizations are not councils at all, but local charities originally set up to provide TB clinics in village halls. Nowadays they have a slightly different character and function depending on where you live, but they should be able to point you to support groups and charities in your area. There is a list of them at <www.acre.org.uk/in-your-area/network-members/>.

Maybe groups are not your thing, in which case you might be more comfortable reading, looking for support online or contacting a relatively anonymous helpline. Some details for these are given in the 'Helpful organizations' section.

Being alone in early recovery is absolutely disastrous.[3]

Twelve Step programmes

For some, the Twelve Step programmes of Alcoholics Anonymous and Narcotics Anonymous are, quite literally, lifesavers. Here is a description of those steps. You can replace the word 'alcohol' with 'drugs' or 'gambling'.

1 We admitted we were powerless over alcohol and that our lives had become unmanageable.
2 Came to believe that a power greater than ourselves could restore us to sanity.
3 Made a decision to turn our will and our lives over to the care of God as we understood Him.

4 Made a searching and fearless moral inventory of ourselves.

5 Admitted to God, to ourselves and to another human being the exact nature of our wrongs.

6 Were entirely ready to have God remove all these defects of character.

7 Humbly asked Him to remove our shortcomings.

8 Made a list of all persons we had harmed and became willing to make amends to them all.

9 Made direct amends to such people wherever possible, except when to do so would injure them or others.

10 Continued to take personal inventory and when we were wrong, promptly admitted it.

11 Sought through prayer and meditation to improve our conscious contact with God as we understood Him, praying only for knowledge of His will for us and the power to carry that out.

12 Having had a spiritual awakening as the result of these steps, we tried to carry this message to alcoholics and to practice these principles in all our affairs.[4]

If this is the first time you have read that list, how did you react to it? If you are not a believer in Christianity, you may find the references to God and prayer rather uncomfortable. You can replace 'God' with 'Higher Power', and 'prayer' with 'meditation' if you wish, and for some people that works. For others, their sense of congruence or authentic self cannot be maintained in the face of this type of language, although for the addict in Chris the religiosity of the language was an excuse to sidestep the challenge to his behaviour that he was being offered.

We can see how the Twelve Step line of progress addresses the problems of 'addictive thinking' identified by Abraham Twerski in *Addictive Thinking* and by Georgia W. in *Don't Let the Bastards Grind You Down*: the self-delusion, the grandiose thinking, the resentment of others, the projections and rationalizations, and most of all the denial. One should not, though, assume that people follow this course of progress one step at a time and – hey presto! – they are recovered! Each person takes his own path, at her own pace, and may need to double-back a few times. For me the antiquated 1930s language suggests also that the Twelve Step approach could be expressed in more up-to-date terms that both take into account recent research into psychological well-being and offer less of a barrier to people of other faiths or none. But a great strength, to my mind, of the Twelve Steps is that by offering access to a sponsor, a safe space and a super-connected group of people with shared experiences, sufferers can *reconnect* and feel the benefit of a worldwide network of millions of people on their side. It can be another 'asset' in your bank of recovery capital.

SMART recovery

If you are dealing with addictive behaviour and find that the Twelve Step programme does not suit you, you might want to look at the SMART programme, which started in 1994 in the USA.[5] As with the Twelve Steps, the programme is based on mutual aid. It accepts that some participants may make use of medication. It is different from the Twelve Steps in its focus on making use of scientific research, which it uses to update its programmes, and in its emphatically non-religious nature. The SMART movement aims to help people:

- build and maintain motivation to live well;
- cope with addictive urges;
- manage thoughts, feelings and behaviours;
- live a balanced life.

People who get involved with the programme are not asked to make a lifelong commitment, as with the Twelve Steps, and can re-engage after leaving if it helps them to deal with problems and relapse. The language of SMART is refreshingly respectful – people are not referred to as 'addicts', 'alcoholics' or 'druggies' at the meetings. The focus is of course on recovery from addiction, though, so in the context of a whole person approach it could be one useful and powerful form of support and personal development among a number of others.

SMART recovery is essentially an abstinence-based approach.

GROW recovery

GROW started in Sydney, Australia, in 1957. Again, it is a mutual aid network: people with common experiences come together to talk and explore what affects them and their learning about recovery. GROW seeks to prevent and help recovery from serious mental illness. Its founders were drawn together by their own experiences of mental ill-health and now GROW has 250 groups in Australia as well as international offices in Ireland, New Zealand, the USA and Trinidad. Not being confined to addiction, it has no specific eligibility criteria and no requirement for any diagnosis. Discussion and meetings are facilitated by experienced participants.

> What made me return to Grow for a second week was knowing that I'd found a haven where I could be with people who understood me and didn't criticize me or judge me. *Jo*[6]

Abstinence

We observed earlier how the debate about whether 'abstinence' or 'harm reduction' is a better approach to helping with addiction has taken on a life of its own that is separate from the care of people who are suffering. In simplistic terms, abstinence-based approaches make 100 per cent freedom from the addictive substance or behaviour either a condition of treatment or the principal indicator of success, or both. Here is what the SMART recovery website says about abstinence:

> What we know is that after one has developed a severe addiction, the simplest, easiest, safest and surest way to keep from repeating past behaviors is total abstinence. This is not to say one may not go through a period of 'day at a time,' or 'week at a time,' or even try a 'harm reduction' approach. Still, if you want the easiest way to minimize the problems in your life, go for abstinence eventually. It actually is much easier to just give it up entirely than punish yourself trying to moderate or control your addictive behavior. Studies have shown that regardless of the method employed to become sober, the number one factor for sobriety success is a permanent commitment to discontinue use permanently; a commitment to abstinence.[7]

It should be noted that sudden and total withdrawal from a substance to which you are severely addicted can in some circumstances be dangerous, even life-threatening, so get help and take advice from people who know what they are talking about.

Harm reduction

'Harm reduction' approaches refer to policies, programmes and practices that 'aim to reduce the harms associated with psycho-active drug use in people unable or unwilling to stop'.[8] Harm reduction has developed a bad name in some quarters because of the practice of 'parking' people addicted to heroin on methadone, a prescribed substitute. Methadone itself is not without risk, and people have expressed fear and frustration about their fate, feeling that their need for help is not being taken seriously and that they are being left to languish indefinitely in a painful limbo of unresolved addiction. The term 'harm reduction' refers to the harm done to others as well as to the person with the addiction as a result of drug misuse, so the basic thinking is that if the problem is not going to go away, then at least it might be possible to reduce the damage it does.

In a whole person approach, you will be working with your medical practitioner or support worker to carefully establish what works *for you*.

Let me give you an example from my personal experience. When I gave up smoking cigarettes, most nicotine substitute products seemed just to make me crave nicotine more – they actually made the problem worse. I had tried gum, patches, self-help books, acupuncture, total abstinence, going on holiday, avoiding the places and friends that tended to trigger me to smoke – you name it. But for some reason nicotine mouth spray enabled me to develop long periods without thinking about having a cigarette, long enough to finally break the habit. It probably helped that I was given the spray free of charge by a terribly nice 'smoking cessation' worker whose office was just around the corner from my house. It was also about the seventh or eighth time I had tried to give up, so by that time I had learned quite a lot about what my particular relapse risks were and I had got better (although not perfect) at avoiding or resisting them. Whatever the reason – who cares? It worked.

Involuntary or coercive treatment

For those who are unable to help themselves, and who are in danger or a danger to others, emergency intervention is both part of the available recovery capital and a potential lifesaver. There will inevitably remain a role for involuntary detention in treatment for such people. It is important for carers to understand this too, as many people are afraid of the stigma attached to a 'section' order, and reluctance to agree to section a person can, as in Chris's case, hasten death. Recovery capital is for friends, family and carers as well as the person struggling with addiction and/or mental health problems.

As we saw from the NHS statistics, around 50,000 people a year are 'sectioned' in the UK. It is a last resort, a lifesaving event for some and hugely resented by others. The quality of care and relationships that people subsequently enjoy (I use the word advisedly) can vary enormously. It is undoubtedly distressing for all concerned, but sometimes also a relief.

What happens, and how treatment or recovery evolve from that point, is determined by an array of factors, including the coping skills of police or social workers, the particular receptiveness of the 'patient', the capabilities of medical staff, the availability of forward treatment options and sometimes the availability of treatment itself. One participant in the RSA research noted that of a group of people who had been sectioned, all bar her had been allocated budget for residential rehab, whereas she had to make do with day care. My own feelings about having to choose, inappropriately and at a moment of utter crisis, whether someone else should be sectioned, was that things should never have got that far, that the help we had asked for should have been offered in full at the point when we first asked for it. I am sure that with more, and more careful, early intervention, a significant proportion of those 'sectioned' or placed on a treatment programme as a result of involvement with the criminal justice system could have been helped sooner, to everyone's benefit.

Learning

You may be familiar with the vogue for getting your 'mental five-a-day' – a public health campaign that urges people to think about ways to build and maintain personal mental well-being in the same way that eating five portions of fruit and vegetables a day helps to maintain physical health. Again, this kind of approach may not help you *solve* the practical, social and economic problems you face, but it can and does help people be more resilient, enabling them to cope, to be more optimistic, more creative, more good-humoured. Not to be sniffed at, therefore. If 'well-being' is the aim, then we need to get an idea of what we mean by the word:

> Sarah Stewart-Brown, professor of public health at the University of Warwick and a wellbeing expert, says that when we talk about mental wellbeing, we mean more than just happiness . . .
>
> 'Feelings of contentment, enjoyment, confidence and engagement with the world are all a part of mental wellbeing. Self-esteem and self-confidence are, too. So is a feeling that you can do the things you want to do. And so are good relationships, which bring joy to you and those around you.
>
> 'Of course, good mental wellbeing does not mean that you never experience feelings or situations that you find difficult. But it does mean that you feel you have the resilience to cope when times are tougher than usual.'
>
> Mental wellbeing can take many different forms, but a useful description is feeling good and functioning well.[9]

The 'five-a-day' approach is a simple checklist of things we can do in our daily lives to give us a boost and replace bad feelings with beneficial ones. Evidence suggests this can really work. Here are the five things.

1 *Connect* – connect with the people around you: your family, friends, colleagues and neighbours. Spend time developing these relationships.
2 *Be active* – you don't have to go to the gym. Go for a walk, go cycling or play a game of football. Find the activity that you enjoy and make it a part of your life.
3 *Keep learning* – learning new skills can give you a sense of achievement and a new confidence. So why not sign up for that cookery course, start learning to play a musical instrument, or figure out how to fix your bike?
4 *Give to others* – even the smallest act can count, whether it's a smile, a thank you or a kind word. Larger acts, such as volunteering at your local community centre, can improve your mental wellbeing and help you build new social networks.
5 *[Take notice]* – be more aware of the present moment, including your feelings and thoughts, your body and the world around you. Some people call this awareness 'mindfulness', and it can

> positively change the way you feel about life and how you
> approach challenges.[10]

Learning is often informal, accidental, serendipitous. It is no less valuable for that. Under the heading of more formal types of 'learning' there are some new and important developments that recognize the value of learning from others with similar experiences and a track record of recovery. We noted in Chapter 2 how important it is to feel understood, and to be able to trust those who are supposed to be supporting us. This idea has been taken a step further in the establishment of 'recovery academies' or 'colleges'. These are places that provide a range of courses for people with mental health or substance misuse problems, their families, carers, volunteers and health care professionals. Courses are free to participants and are jointly designed and facilitated by experts by experience and experts by profession. Courses may be one day, or may last a few weeks or longer, and enable people to improve their understanding of mental health issues, learn ways to manage a condition, or simply connect with other people and learn something new. One such 'college' in Manchester offers courses in the categories of 'Lived Experience, Supporting Recovery, Developing Knowledge and Life Skills and Getting Involved with the Academy. The range of courses available each term will vary as the academy responds to the demands of its students.'[11]

Under these broad headings there are a range of learning opportunities, such as creative writing (an activity for which there is a growing body of evidence to suggest the mental health benefits) and 'making advance decisions'. Participants are free to propose new courses if they feel there may be a benefit to people in recovery. The courses take place across the city in accessible places like community centres, hospitals and theatres.

Learning styles

It is a common experience, and one shared by many people who do not feel they have a mental health problem, to find that formal or structured learning like this is unappealing. This is often rooted in our experiences of school. The world of learning has changed, however, and as well as looking at learning opportunities with an open mind and being prepared to give things a try, it is worth understanding a little about how we as individuals best learn. You may have heard about 'learning styles' or 'learning preferences' – if you are able to know a little about how you personally best process information and new ideas, which may well be different from the way I or the person next to you does it, then you will be able to focus on activities that not only suit you and your recovery best but are also *more enjoyable*. Right now you are reading a book, and for many of us that is a common way of learning something – it is my *preferred* way of learning – but there are many other ways of taking in and making use of new information or acquiring new skills.

Professor Howard Gardner, an American educational psychologist, has developed a way to define people's different preferences, and his work has been profoundly influential.[12] He argues that traditional IQ testing is only one, somewhat limited, way of assessing people's mental capabilities. In essence, his research suggests that there are a range of 'intelligences' or perceptual types that we all have to some degree, but the balance and emphasis of these varies greatly from person to person. See if any of these rings a bell for you:

- *linguistic*: a preference for reading, writing, verbalizing
- *logical/mathematical*: a preference for patterns, puzzles, numbering, sequences
- *musical*: a preference for rhythm, melody, lyricism, hearing and listening
- *bodily/kinaesthetic*: a preference for movement, physicality and learning by doing
- *visual/spatial*: a preference for drawing, diagrams, illustration, film, colour
- *interpersonal*: a preference for dialogue, conversation, sharing learning with others
- *intrapersonal*: a preference for solitary thinking, inward reflection, contemplation.

It is fun to assess your own learning preferences, and you can do this for free at <www.businessballs.com/howardgardnermultiple intelligences.htm>. This self-testing technique helps you find out which are your particular strengths, and may also help you see why some types of learning don't suit you so well.

Here are some ideas, organized by learning preference, about the activities that might work for you when it comes to getting your mental five-a-day. This is just a brief overview and you may have better ideas. You could brainstorm with people in your recovery network to see whether your preference is:

- *linguistic*: reading books, magazines, websites; writing a journal; emails and letter-writing; mnemonics (using the initial letters of things to remember them all, e.g. Every Good Boy Deserves Football – EGBDF – is a way of remembering the notes of the treble clef in music);
- *logical/mathematical*: playing games, creating patterns, doing puzzles, numbering, creating sequences, coding;
- *musical*: playing music; listening to music while learning; using music, rhyme or songs to remember things;
- *bodily/kinaesthetic*: playing sport, dancing, walking, making things;
- *visual/spatial*: drawing, diagrams, illustration, watching videos, using colour;
- *interpersonal*: classes and workshops, dialogue, conversation, debate, sharing learning with others (e.g. walking and talking);
- *intrapersonal*: keeping a diary, reading, quiet reflection, memorizing, mindfulness.

These preferences can shift over our lifetimes as we develop and change. They are not a fixed way of telling you how you are or how you must be, simply a way of gaining some helpful insight into your own learning and development, so that it is a more productive and enjoyable process for you.

Work and money

Difficulties with finding or sustaining work, and with money, can (obviously) compound psychological suffering of all kinds. Indeed, problems with work and money can themselves be triggers for mental health problems. As with other aspects of recovery, however, support is available. The quality and accessibility of that support varies from place to place, but it *is* there. Many of these forms of help have taken a battering from the austerity cuts, especially in the charitable sector, and people may have to be patient in waiting for an appointment, but services remain and they are invaluable. The National Debt Helpline, for example (see 'Helpful organizations') is a first port of call if you are struggling with debt. They can provide advice and compassionate, non-judgemental and common-sense support. They can also liaise on your behalf with people you owe money to. Having enough money to get by is a challenge for many people at the best of times, so the debt helpline can also help with budgeting for the future.

When it comes to work and earning, we may want to go back to Bruce Alexander to remind ourselves that we do not always have as much power over these things as we would like. A great deal of what happens to us is governed by great forces beyond our individual control – but that is not to say that there is nothing we can do. Speaking with someone who had been made redundant twice in three years, and who was afflicted by severe depression, I was struck by how much of his identity was wrapped up in work. He did a number of things to try to boost his mood, including playing in a band, avoiding stressful situations, and accepting (eventually) support from a counsellor and prescription antidepressants. These appear to have provided some benefit, but the real catalyst for major improvement was getting a new job. He treated job-hunting as a job in itself, working on it from nine to five for over a year and experiencing multiple rejections. The job he was finally offered paid half what he had previously earned, and was below his skill and experience level – but it was meaningful work that suited his values, in an empathetic environment. And at the end of the day he can switch off and go home. It was the right job, in other words, and he found himself able to live with the drop in status. It can help to take a step down like this if your job is making you ill.

If you want to stay in your current job, if you have one, then building your recovery capital should include ensuring recuperation outside of work, support that works for you, whether that is a cup of tea with a friend, quality time with the kids, a walk in the woods, a trip to the gym or library, or time to have a massage and relax. It's good, if you can, to plan these times ahead so you have something to look forward to. Make sure you won't be interrupted.

> Every person needs to take one day away. A day in which one consciously separates the past from the future. Jobs, lovers, family, employers and friends can all exist one day without any

one of us, and if our egos permit us to confess, they could exist eternally in our absence . . .

Each person deserves a day away in which no problems are confronted, no solutions searched for. Each of us needs to withdraw from the cares which will not withdraw from us. We need hours of aimless wandering or spates of time sitting on park benches, observing the mysterious world of ants and the canopy of treetops.

If we step away for a time we are not, as many may think and some will accuse, being irresponsible, but rather we are preparing ourselves to more ably perform our duties and discharge our obligations.[13]

Maybe work is not feasible for you, or not at the moment, but you still want something constructive to do, or to have a regular opportunity to connect with other people. There will be many volunteering opportunities locally, in charities, community groups or the NHS for example, where your life experience and empathy will be priceless. Try your local voluntary services centre for information, or contact the group or organization that you are most interested in directly. *Be clear with them and yourself as to what is a realistic amount of time and commitment for you.* Do not over-stretch yourself.

In order to make sure any work or volunteering you tackle does not leave you worse off financially, do seek advice from your Citizens' Advice Bureau or benefits advice centre: they have regularly updated software that can help you navigate the maze of ever-changing rules and regulations.

I will not specifically address the question of state benefits and rules for people out of work or on a low income here, because the regulations change so often and, despite the best efforts of many professional and compassionate individuals, the general tenor of political rhetoric in these areas is distastefully punitive. I worked on a project helping people in rural areas facing barriers to employment – including health problems, disability, long-term unemployment, lone parenthood, caring commitments, isolation, a lack of work skills, a recent exit from the criminal justice system – get back into work, and I was struck by how well-informed and caring *some* employees of the Department of Work and Pensions actually are (though I am sure they are not all so). In particular

I remember one young woman who delayed referring disabled people to a programme run by a large private company because she was worried that its staff simply did not have the relevant expertise or humanity. The senior management of the state, private sector and charitable organizations responsible for implementing changes in government policy, however, have ploughed on regardless, impervious to challenge. It was not at all clear to me that what was happening was not in some way designed to punish people for being ill or poor. In theory the programme could have been interesting and flexible enough to adapt to individual circumstances – perfect for recovery. In practice it became, as far as I could see, a way not to sustain people but to transfer money and responsibility away from the taxpayer and into the coffers of unaccountable organizations. This is a personal view.

Whole person recovery: a reminder

The Mental Health Foundation gives an appealing description of how to think about the recovery process. Recovery, it says,

- provides a holistic view of mental illness that focuses on the person, not just his or her symptoms;
- includes the belief that recovery from severe mental illness is possible;
- is a journey rather than a destination;
- does not necessarily mean getting back to where you were before;
- happens in 'fits and starts' and, like life, has many ups and downs;
- calls for optimism and commitment from all concerned;
- is profoundly influenced by people's expectations and attitudes;
- requires a well-organized system of support from family, friends or professionals;
- requires services to embrace new and innovative ways of working;
- aims to help people with mental health problems to look beyond mere survival and existence, encouraging them to move forward, set new goals and do things and develop relationships that give their lives meaning;
- emphasizes that, while people may not have full control over their symptoms, they can have full control over their lives.

Recovery is not about 'getting rid' of problems. It is about seeing beyond people's mental health problems, recognizing and fostering their abilities, interests and dreams.[14]

And here is the RSA's recovery cycle again, with a few suggestions as to how to deal with each step.

- *The baggage*: finding ways to manage past feelings and experiences. Options include asking for help from professionals such as GPs and counsellors. Keep a journal of your feelings. Join a support group where you can share your feelings with others in the same boat. Read. Take up creative activities.
- *Breaking routines*: developing skills and capabilities for the future. Learn something new. Connect with new people. Change your daily routine (or introduce one). Find ways to put difficult people and places behind you. Have fun in ways that do you good.
- *Treatment*: formal and informal services and support. Find a medical practitioner or support worker that you trust. Ask for advice from other people in recovery. Tell the professionals what works and what doesn't. Turn up to your appointments. Join a support group. Research your condition. Find a mentor.
- *Making a plan*: formal and informal coping strategies. Create regular time to rest and recuperate. Fit your mental five-a-day into your plan for the week. Find out about yourself and what works for you. Set yourself short-term goals (but don't use them to beat yourself up). Dream and create a long-term goal. Make a list of all the people and organizations that can help you.
- *The rest of my life*: getting well and staying well. Live in the moment – take notice and enjoy the little things. Keep learning. Have fun. Be kind. Celebrate your achievements, no matter how small. Connect with like-minded people. Avoid triggers and bad places or people. Take time out to reflect.

Stick this list on your fridge (or some other suitable place). Take good care of yourself. Prepare to do well and also to fail sometimes. Life goes on.

Moving on

Making the decision to change can be daunting. Success is not guaranteed. Relapses are possible. You may lose things that have become a major, if not *the* major, part of your life. The barriers may be easier to overcome than you think, or *much* more difficult. Breaking the routine and doing things anew is a battle that people who haven't done it might not understand. You may have to live with being imperfect and failing from time to time. Imagine! Motivations will be as different as they can be:

I'll give up by looking at people and thinking that ain't me. I don't want to end up like that.[15]

I have my plan but then I need more of a fix because it has a hold of me that means I'm creating more of a downer, and then eventually I lose the plan and hit rock bottom.[16]

Friends and family. They are the ones that started me out.

When I got clean it wasn't the drugs I missed, it was the environment. I missed skulking about . . . So I reckon the scene would be the one to break.[17]

My kids were totally disgusted with me.[18]

Early recovery for a lot of people is, 'It's just for today.'[19]

Well, I fucked up and it's perfectly right for people to be sceptical. I know I've got work to do to regain trust.[20]

Creating a whole new you out of the existing one, learning from the pain of the past and replacing it with something safer and more enjoyable, are bound not to be easy. It is tempting to look backwards and think what you might be giving up:

I'm a better person on drugs. Without them I wouldn't be sitting here right now; I'd get angry. I don't talk at all. I'm just no fun to be around unless I've either taken something or drunk something.[21]

The power of dope comes from the first time you do it. It's a deep memory disease. People know the first time is important, but mostly they're confused about why. Some think addiction is nostalgia for the first mind-blowing time. They think the addict's problem is wanting something that happened a long time ago to come back. That's not it at all. The addict's problem is that something that happened a long time ago never goes away. To me, the white tops are still as new and fresh as the first time.[22]

According to his interviewer, the journalist Decca Aitkenhead, recovering plagiarist Johann Hari says his new life 'makes him happier and healthier than his old one ever could'.[23] It is a common story – just very hard to believe when you haven't got there yet.

Recovery does not involve denying your experience or abandoning what you know. It is not about seeking perfection – that is bound to end in failure. It is about facing things, evolving and moving on to a better place, at a pace that works – to live the rest of your life. To give a modest example, when I left home at 18 I had developed an extreme over-reactiveness to the sound of banging doors. Truly, I would leap out my skin and burst into a sweat, even at something that was not especially loud. As I write this I can feel my skin prickle at the thought.

But these days I understand what is going on: when someone has been through a traumatic experience, reminders of aspects of that experience can trigger what is called 'hyper-vigilance'. Our 'fight-or-flight' adrenaline response to a perceived threat or danger goes into overdrive, and effectively becomes a permanent part of our toolkit for reacting to the world. In my case it is relatively minor, an aural association with the violent home I grew up in. The effects are intrusive and unpleasant, but momentary. However for, say, a soldier returning from active duty in a war zone, or a paramedic dealing with the aftermath of car crashes, this can be a debilitating condition that they may want to deal with quite specifically in order to feel able to go forward to a more comfortable place in their life. My experience means that at least to some degree I 'get' what it is that others affected by hyper-vigilance feel. I would rather not feel it, but it is useful to know and gives me insight. We do not have to throw the baby out with the bath water.

> Something can be gained, retrospectively . . . there is a 'glimpse of timelessness, that little chip of immortality that lies at the centre of the disease and recovery.[24]

Hope comes in many forms. Ways to remind ourselves of what can be achieved are everywhere, if we take notice. In Liverpool, Glasgow, Brighton and other cities, people celebrate with an annual 'recovery walk', hundreds of people literally taking recovery to the streets in affirmation and recognition.

When the workshop participants I worked with were asked to define recovery, these were the most important elements they came up with:

- physical well-being
- self-care

- self-awareness
- state of mind
- learning to live
- it's thriving not surviving.

> Though we live in a world that dreams of ending
> That always seems about to give in
> Something will not acknowledge conclusion
> Insists that we forever begin.[25]

Helpful organizations

In an ideal world I would like to ask everyone who has read this book to share the resources, assets or 'recovery capital' that they would recommend to others. That is not very practical, however, so inevitably what you will find here is a mixture of things from which you can take whatever fits and works for you. Look over this section and the next and treat them as a starting point. It is worth noting that Mind, Rethink and the Mental Health Foundation, as well as NHS Choices, all offer information on their websites about specific mental health conditions such as anxiety, depression, bipolar disorder, schizophrenia and addiction, as well as links to further support. A few organizations even have useful apps that you can install on your phone. Information in this section is organized as follows:

- websites, principally of support and advice organizations
- NHS and private/charitable health services.

Your number one recovery asset, though, is your own natural ability to recover, *given the right circumstances*. The next most important asset on the list is probably genuine human connection with *people you know and trust*. So these sections are intended to help support you in creating those things. As you go through them, look back again at the RSA's summary of the recovery journey (see p. 68) and pick out those ideas that you feel may work for you as you plot your way.

Websites

Al-Anon

www.al-anonuk.org.uk

Al-Anon is an international organization with over 800 groups in the UK and Ireland. The groups are for the friends and families of alcoholics (and drug users), and are run along similar lines to other Twelve Step programmes such as Alcoholics Anonymous and Narcotics Anonymous.

Alcoholics Anonymous

www.alcoholics-anonymous.org.uk

AA is the world's biggest peer-led organization for people affected by problematic alcohol use. As well as a helpline and other forms of support for people at any stage of their recovery journey (or even just thinking about it), the AA website offers support for professionals and a search facility to find local groups.

Bipolar UK

www.bipolaruk.org.uk

This is the national charity dedicated to supporting people affected by bipolar disorder and to helping them take control of their lives.

CALM: The Campaign Against Living Miserably

www.thecalmzone.net

They say: 'CALM is a registered charity, which exists to prevent male suicide in the UK. In 2013, male suicide accounts for 78% of all suicides and is the single biggest cause of death in men aged 20–45 in England and Wales.' CALM offers support to men of any age who are down or in crisis via a helpline and their website. It also hosts the Suicide Bereavement Support partnership, 'which includes Cruse, If U Care Share, Papyrus, SoBS and the Samaritans amongst others . . . This partnership aims to ensure that everyone bereaved or affected by suicide is offered and receives timely and appropriate support.'

Central government

www.gov.uk

This is the online home for official advice and information about anything to do with central government. For example, if you want to work out how different hours of work or changing your job might affect any entitlement to tax credit payments from HM Revenue & Customs, you can go to <www.gov.uk/tax-credits-calculator>.

The Citizens' Advice Bureau

www.citizensadvice.org.uk

The CAB, which has branches all over the UK and many of which are run by volunteers, helps people solve work, money and legal problems by providing well-informed, confidential advice, information and guidance. Their online advice guide is at <www.adviceguide.org.uk/>.

The national helpline number and the location of your local branch can be found at <www.citizensadvice.org.uk/index/get advice.htm>.

The Depression Alliance

www.depressionalliance.org

The Depression Alliance aims to help people by tackling the loneliness and isolation of depression. In particular they run the Friends in Need scheme for people affected by depression or supporting someone who is, which enables people to talk online or meet up in local groups.

Drugscope

www.drugscope.org.uk

Drugscope provides research, training and support for professionals working in the drug sector and is a leading centre of expertise on drug use.

Family Lives

www.familylives.org.uk

Family Lives is a national charity providing non-judgemental help and support for a range of common troubles that families may find themselves dealing with, including arguments, school or workplace bullying, and worries about teenagers. They also offer online parenting courses to help busy parents learn new tips and coping strategies.

The Fredericks Foundation

www.fredericksfoundation.org

Set up in 2001 by Paul Barry-Walsh, the Fredericks Foundation seeks to help those who would like to stop being dependent on benefits set up their own businesses. It also assists existing companies in need of finance when they are unable to obtain funds from their banks.

The Mental Health Foundation

www.mentalhealth.org.uk

The Mental Health Foundation is an advice, research and campaigning organization: 'We are working for an end to mental ill-health and the inequalities that face people experiencing mental distress, living with learning disabilities or reduced mental capacity.'

The MHF website has some helpful information on the experiences of black people and those from other ethnic minorities, in relation to both mental health and to services and treatment.

Mind

www.mind.org.uk

Mind is an important national charity whose motto is 'we won't give up until everyone experiencing a mental health problem gets both support and respect'. In many local areas they provide services like groups and meetings, information, advice, and representation and advocacy (i.e. speaking up for you) with councils, the health service and other official bodies.

Mind Out

www.mindout.org.uk

'MindOut is a mental health service run by and for lesbians, gay men, bisexual and transgender people. Based in Brighton and Hove, we provide local services as well as a number of national initiatives. We provide advice, information, advocacy, a peer support group programme, well-being activities and events and a food & allotment project.'

Narcotics Anonymous

ukna.org

NA is run along similar lines to AA. This what they say: 'N.A. is a non-profit fellowship or society of men and women for whom drugs had become a major problem. We are recovering addicts who meet regularly to help each other stay clean. This is a program of complete abstinence from all drugs. There is only ONE requirement for membership, the desire to stop using. We suggest that you keep an open mind and give yourself a break.'

The National Debt Helpline

www.nationaldebtline.org

This helpline provides online and telephone help to deal with debt, bills and budgeting.

Recovery-focused sites

www.recovery.org
www.smartrecovery.org.uk

Relate

www.relate.org.uk

The UK's biggest provider of relationship advice and counselling. Every year they help 'over a million people of all ages, backgrounds and sexual orientation'. Services include confidential counselling for couples and singles, sex therapy and a range of self-help tools, such as books and self-assessment quizzes. Charges, where they exist, can be flexible to take account of your circumstances. Relate also provides relationship skills training for professionals and volunteers in the corporate, public and charity sectors.

Rethink Mental Illness

www.rethink.org

Another big national charity, Rethink 'provide[s] a range of services nationally including advocacy, carer support, crisis services and more'. There are helpline numbers on the website for people suffering mental health difficulties and also for carers and family members.

The Royal College of Psychiatrists

www.rcpsych.ac.uk

This is the website of the professional body that represents the 'medical' end of the mental health services spectrum. They rightly point out that most mental health problems do not need a psychiatrist. As well as information for professionals, the site also has some useful resources for the general public, including an explanation of local mental health services.

The Samaritans

www.samaritans.org

Famously, the Samaritans provide a free, non-judgemental listening service, 24 hours a day, 365 days a year. 'If something is troubling you, get in touch. We help you talk things through. We keep everything confidential. We are not a religious organization.'

The Trussell Trust

www.trusselltrust.org

The Trussell Trust describes its mission as 'restoring dignity and reviving hope'. It runs community projects to tackle poverty and isolation, and the website has a map of food banks across the UK.

Turning Point

www.turning-point.co.uk

Turning Point is a 'social enterprise, providing specialist and integrated services which focus on improving lives and communities across mental health, learning disability, substance misuse, primary care, the criminal justice system and employment'. In many areas the organization provides services in alliance with the NHS and local councils.

Women's Aid

www.womensaid.org.uk

Women's Aid is a national charity working to end what is euphemistically known as 'domestic abuse' against women and children. Abuse can include physical violence, psychological control and coercion, sexual abuse and financial abuse. These are all under-reported, and the last especially so. Many women affected by substance misuse, mental ill-health and/or by entanglement with the police and criminal justice system are also affected by domestic abuse. The website contains lots of very useful information on a range of topics from children to immigration and from the police to dealing with perpetrators. They are very experienced at dealing with the safety concerns of women seeking help and have a telephone helpline. They can point you safely and quickly to the nearest source of help, although local and national government budget cuts often affect the availability of, for example, refuge accommodation.

YoungMinds

www.youngminds.org.uk

This organization provides 'straight talk and honest answers' for young people wanting to know about mental health. 'YoungMinds is the UK's leading charity committed to improving the emotional well-being and mental health of children and young people.' They provide services for children and young people, for parents and carers, and for professionals.

The NHS and local mental health services

The National Health Service

Your GP

The first port of call for many people seeking help or advice from the NHS will be their general practitioner (GP), but at the time of writing getting a GP appointment was becoming increasingly difficult to accomplish (last time I had to make an appointment it took me eight attempts to get through by phone). Hopefully this is just a temporary aberration and the powers-that-be will get around to restoring the NHS we know and love. Your GP is obliged to offer *confidential* support and can refer you to a range of specialist services, including addiction programmes and the local mental health team, where you should be able to get an assessment of your needs and some form of treatment plan if appropriate. The time this takes and the level of support varies enormously, so you may wish to have other forms of back-up available as well, for example from one of the charities listed above. If you are employed, your GP can certify your absence from work on health grounds so that you can qualify for state benefits if necessary and your employer can reclaim some sick pay from HMRC.

Do note that in some areas you can refer yourself to addiction services and do not have to go through your GP.

NHS Choices

www.nhs.uk/Pages/HomePage.aspx

NHS choices gives comprehensive advice on health conditions and provides a search facility to help you find services near you. NHS Choices has some good information and links on living well, boosting your mental well-being and finding care and support, including advice on financial support for carers, getting a care plan and planning for your future needs.

Your local mental health services

At the time of writing, these were going through the latest phase of restructuring and reorganization demanded by politicians. Get advice from friends, your GP or the local NHS trust on what is available to you. People working in community mental health teams might include mental health workers, psychiatrists, community psychiatric nurses (CPNs), social workers, occupational therapists, clinical psychologists, pharmacists, assertive outreach workers and people attached to the Child and Adolescent Mental Health Service (CAMHS). There may also be counsellors working in a range of ways, including offering Cognitive Behavioural Therapy, Person-Centred Therapy, Psychodynamic Therapy, Integrative Therapy, family support and trauma counselling. Do not worry if you are not clear on the differences between these approaches – research shows that what matters most and makes counselling or psychotherapy most effective is the quality of the relationship between you and your counsellor. So trust your instincts.

In-patient rehabilitation

'Rehab' in other words. Provision across the country is patchy and waiting times can test patience, but NHS rehab does exist. This is how the Central and North West London NHS Foundation Trust describes its rehab services:

> Inpatient rehabilitation is provided for people who have complex mental health problems and where previous placements have been unable to meet their needs.
> There is a range of services to meet different service user needs and levels of support. The services provide a homely environment for people with mental health problems.
> Qualified and experienced teams support service users to develop the necessary skills for independent living, including practical skills, mental health management and feeling prepared psychologically.

Service users and their relatives or carers are encouraged to work with staff to draw up a programme of care. The programme includes learning or relearning life skills, a range of group and individual therapies, activities and access to leisure, education and employment opportunities in the community.[1]

Referral processes and locations are very variable across the country, so in the first instance contact your GP or local mental health trust, if you think this might be for you.

Drug and Alcohol Action Teams (DAATs)

Sometimes embedded in local 'recovery partnerships', these are specialist interdisciplinary teams dealing with the challenges created by substance misuse, including health care, homelessness, family support and skills training. Oxfordshire DAAT describes itself as 'Commissioning drug and alcohol treatment and support services for young people, adults, families and carers throughout Oxfordshire' (www.oxfordshiredaat.org)

'Commissioning' means deciding (generally on the basis of some form of local consultation and in-house expertise) what services should be available in a given place and providing the money to pay for them. The DAAT may also provide a formal bridge or communications link between different services – essential to any kind of whole person approach that personalizes care and support according to the needs of individuals, rather than creating a 'one size fits all' service that sets people up to fail.

The National Treatment Agency

This was the section of the NHS that until 2013 managed substance and alcohol misuse services specifically, at the national level. The NTA has now been merged into . . .

Public Health England

The PHE website contains links to:

- emergency contacts
- health and well-being resources
- health protection A to Z
- data and knowledge gateway
- contacts: PHE regions and local centres.

It is part of the argument of this book that addiction and mental suffering are major social and public health problems (as opposed to a problem for individuals alone), so let us hope the disappearance of the NTA into Public Health England turns out to be a good thing and not the beginning of the end of the recovery movement in the NHS.

The National Institute for Health and Care Excellence (NICE)

You have probably heard of 'NICE Guidelines'. These are the official, evidence-based rules issued by NICE to guide NHS staff in the diagnosis and treatment of a vast array of medical conditions. If, like me, you are keen to understand how and why doctors make certain decisions, these rules are publicly available. You can search online for information about your condition or circumstances at <www.nice.org.uk>. For example, Guidance Note 100 is *Alcohol Use Disorders: Diagnosis and clinical management of alcohol-related physical complications* (<www.nice.org.uk/guidance/cg100>).

Charitable and private health services

In addition to those activities noted above, charitable and private sector organizations may be contracted by local government or the NHS to provide, for example, rehab services, and they may also provide these for people who have access to the financial resources to pay for health care. Here are two examples:

The BAC O'Connor Centre

www.bacandoconnor.co.uk

This award-winning rehab centre, often cited as an example of 'best practice', is run by Noreen Oliver, the founder and chief executive, who used her own experiences of addiction and recovery in establishing the centre in 1998. Residents are asked to make a very modest contribution to food costs of around £25 per week.

The Priory

www.priorygroup.com

At the other end of the spectrum, the Priory group of hospitals describes itself as 'Europe's leading provider of rehabilitation services' and has 275 hospitals, clinics and schools across the UK. Services are not cheap but can sometimes be paid for by employers' or personal health insurance policies. If you do have health insurance that will cover this, you should ensure that it will pay for the full length of your stay. If you need to stay for six months but your insurers will only pay for one, you may want to consider NHS provision instead – you may even find that some of the staff work in both places. The Priory Group do though point to their 'success' rates in helping people into recovery as being better than those of the NHS. That may be for a number of reasons including, possibly, that more affluent clients also have greater access to other forms of recovery capital such as secure housing, a regular income, stable social networks, learning and leisure opportunities.

Other resources for recovery

Leisure and learning

It may be that you will want to move away from harmful people and activities, and give your time and attention to things that are good for you and enjoyable. From cooking to beach volleyball, from meditation to juggling, there is bound to be something that appeals. Here are some suggestions:

Film/video

A search online will reveal any number of affecting and insightful videos related to recovery. This one of Carl Rogers counselling a client – worth watching if you want to see what *real* listening is like – can be found at <www.youtube.com/watch?v=24d-FEptYj8> (45 minutes, filmed in 1965 in the USA).

The NIIS is increasingly offering fixed-term courses of cognitive behavioural therapy (CBT); some people report it to be helpful, while others think it addresses symptoms but not causes or any need for deep, underlying change. This video gives an example of 'brief CBT' that shows what it can be like: <www.youtube.com/watch?v=fCZpUIEUsys> (3 minutes 20 seconds, UK).

And here is an example of a session of counselling for depression based on 'mindfulness': <www.youtube.com/watch?v=0mrgqXoQI80> (12 minutes, USA).

Joining a film club can open your eyes and connect you with people. Learning to make your own films or improving your photography skills can give a focus to your natural creativity: perhaps you can create a visual record of significant events and places in your recovery? Or, if that is a bit earnest for you, maybe you could develop an interest in photographing landscape, faces or sport.

If you like the idea of this but don't feel confident, try looking at <learnbasicphotography.com>.

Reading

Reading as part of your recovery falls into two categories: reading about your condition and about the associated strategies for coping and improving your well-being, and reading for pleasure. Perhaps surprisingly, it may be the second category that is the more powerful. You may be able to think now of a book that has changed your life or the way you understand something.

Reading is not for everyone, but there is a growing body of evidence to suggest that reading produces measurable benefits to mood, empathy and cognitive function.[1] In a sense, it does not really matter whether these benefits arise from distraction, peacefulness, the imaginative work that goes on when we read, the 'work' that reading makes us do, something scientific to do with neurones and brain networks, or some combination of these – if it works, then it is a very cheap or even free activity.

And reading is not a single activity: reading silently is rather different from reading aloud, and both offer benefits. One of the great pleasures of my week is reading to groups of older people staying in respite care after a period of illness in hospital. The book *A Little, Aloud: An anthology of prose and poetry for reading aloud to someone you care for*, edited by Angela Macmillan (London: Chatto and Windus, 2010) is a good starting point.

Learning to recite poems by heart is another beneficial form of reading. Joining a reading group is a way of using books to make and enjoy human connection and discussion. Visiting the library is a good way to get out of the house, get a change of scenery and get some new ideas. My excellent local library ran projects with arts charity the Reading Agency called Reading Well: Books on Prescription and Mood-Boosting Books, and published a list of books recommended by local people.[2] Search for 'Brighton and Hove Mood-Boosting Books' or go to: <www.brighton-hove.gov.uk/sites/brighton-hove.gov.uk/files/Mood%20Boost%20Winners%20Poster%20B%26H.pdf>.

There is an endless supply of books for all moods and purposes. Speak with your local librarian or bookseller to get some recommendations. As you would expect from someone who has a preference for learning by reading, I have ample reading resources. Here are some recommended book lists I prepared for an event at an arts festival:

Fiction – mood-enhancing books for adults

Alain-Fournier, *Le Grand Meaulnes*

Maya Angelou, *I Know Why the Caged Bird Sings*
Louis de Bernières, *Captain Corelli's Mandolin*
Gerald Durrell, *My Family and Other Animals*
Winifred Foley, *A Child of the Forest*
Joanne Harris, *Chocolat*
Philip Hensher, *Scenes from Early Life*
Laurie Lee, *Cider with Rosie*
Toni Morrison, *Song of Solomon*
Tom Robbins, *Even Cowgirls Get the Blues*
Will Self, *A Quantity Theory of Insanity*

Understanding adversity

Chimamanda Ngozi Adichie, *Half of a Yellow Sun*
Shalom Auslander, *Hope: A Tragedy*
Charles Dickens, *Great Expectations*
Valerie Martin, *Property*
Andrew O'Hagan, *Be Near Me*
Gillian Slovo, *Ice Road*
William Styron, *Darkness Visible*
Alice Walker, *The Color Purple*
Edmund White, *The Farewell Symphony*

Caring, bereavement, trauma, attachment and loss

Douglas Dunn, *Elegies (Poems)*
Patricia Ferguson, *The Midwife's Daughter*
Margaret Forster, *Have the Men had Enough?*
Alexander Masters, *Stuart: A Life Backwards*
Blake Morrison, *And When Did You Last See Your Father?*
Toni Morrison, *Beloved*
Bernhard Schlink, *The Reader*
Kamila Shamsie, *Burnt Shadows*
Anne Tyler, *The Beginner's Goodbye*
Jeanette Winterson, *Why Be Happy When You Could Be Normal?*

Books engaging with the world around us

Diane Ackerman, *A Natural History of the Senses*
Peter Ackroyd, *Thames: Sacred River*
Ronald Blythe, *Akenfield*
Roger Deakin, *Waterlog*

Olivia Laing, *To the River*
Richard Mabey, *The Perfumier and the Stinkhorn*
Robert Macfarlane, *The Old Ways*
Caryl Phillips, *Atlantic Sound*
Iain Sinclair, *London Orbital*

Fiction – books for young people on serious themes

(as recommended by Leila, aged 12)
Malorie Blackman, *Noughts and Crosses* (pacey story dealing with gangs and racism)
Anne Cassidy, *Looking for JJ* (dealing with child murder, identity and secrets)
John Green, *The Fault in Our Stars* (cancer, sadness)
Scott Westerfeld, *Uglies* (themes of self-image, belonging and rule-breaking)

Non-fiction – self-help books for young people

(as recommended by East Sussex Libraries)
Fiona Bleach, *Everybody is Different* (for young people with a sibling with autism)
Dawn Huebner, *What to Do When You Worry Too Much*
Charlotte Moore, *George and Sam* (memoir by a parent of an autistic child)
Kate Cohen-Posey, *How to Handle Bullies, Teasers and Other Meanies*

Books recommended by other event participants

Angela Carter, *Wise Children*: 'This was my favourite author's last book, written when she knew she was dying. Because she was ill I had to wait a long time for it, which made it all the more precious. It's full of warmth, humour and humanity, both literary and a cracking read.'
Any novel by Jasper Fforde: 'I can recommend any of these, I just love them. Even the grammar is alive!'
Stella Gibbons, *Cold Comfort Farm*: 'It made me laugh and gave me immense pleasure.'
Susan Jeffers, *Feel the Fear and Do It Anyway*: 'This book helped me deal with anxiety at a time in my life when there was no other source of help available. I learned to live with it and move on.'

James W. Jones, *In the Middle of this Road We Call Our Life*: 'It's on spirituality and psychoanalysis. It affirmed my beliefs. Reading it was like a game of Tetris.'

Erich Maria Remarque, *All Quiet on the Western Front*: 'I read it young and again later. It gave me validation, helped me form my opinions and gave me strength.'

Sathnam Sanghera, *The Boy with the Topknot*: 'It's about secrets and lies. It made the 1960s tangible for me with its detail, description and humour.'

Nigel Slater, *Toast*: 'It's about home and family life, simple and descriptive. It resonated with my own upbringing.'

Here is a poetry anthology that is good to dip into too: *Staying Alive: Real poems for unreal times*, edited by Neil Astley (Tarset: Bloodaxe Books, 2002).

Music

Listening to music, playing – or learning – can have life-sustaining power. Singing is often said to boost endorphin production in the brain, and that may not just be speculation. A pilot project run by Brighton Health and Wellbeing Centre and Brighton and Sussex Medical School reported not only that people found breathing, movement and general health improved as a result of taking part in a singing group, but that around 80 per cent also made new friends and felt happier. Rhythmix, a music organization in the south east of England, was given funding by the Amy Winehouse Foundation to work with young people. Mark Davyd, CEO of Rhythmix, said:

> Music is an amazing tool by which we can reach out and offer support at a challenging time . . . These projects will enable them to express their emotions and their concerns through their own music and lyrics, something that is incredibly important to us and the Foundation.[3]

The Foundation was set up by Mitch Winehouse, father of Amy, the singer who died at the age of 27, to work to prevent the harmful effects of drug and alcohol misuse on young people.

Art

The benefits of visual arts activity (painting, collage, drawing, printing, etc.) in clinical and therapeutic settings like hospitals and residential care are well established: it is possible to train and practise within the NHS as an art therapist. But art need not be so formal or serious. Any number of local art groups and courses are available in many villages, towns and cities, where you can try different activities and find something that suits you (this is about fun, and both developing your expression and making human connections, so look for something where you will enjoy the atmosphere too). Local further education colleges can often offer free or very cheap courses to people on a low income.

If you don't want to get messy, you might enjoy going to galleries and museums – perhaps team up with a friend or two. You can get some ideas and look up artworks in collections local to you at <www.bbc.co.uk/arts/yourpaintings>. Click on the 'Galleries and Collections' tab to search by location.

There are limitless other creative pursuits that can boost your confidence and well-being: drama, creative writing, jewellery making, carpentry, sculpture, pottery . . . You don't have to be a genius, just find something to enjoy.

Sport

The relationship between regular physical activity and mental well-being is established. Most local authorities have initiatives in hand to encourage people to do more team or individual sport and more physical activity generally. By contacting your local council or leisure centre you should be able to get plenty of information about a full range of activities to suit your level and location. You don't need to buy loads of fancy kit, or pay to join a gym or a formal club (although if that works for you, fine). Park runs are common all over the country:

> Parkrun organise free, weekly, 5km timed runs around the world. They are open to everyone, free, and are safe and easy to take part in. These events take place in pleasant parkland surroundings and we encourage people of every ability to take part; from those taking their first steps in running to Olympians; from juniors to those with more experience; we welcome you all.

See <www.parkrun.org.uk>.

Regular walking is fantastic for heart and mind: you can set yourself a small target and then work your way up to something more ambitious. My local walks are in the South Downs National Park, where I get the benefit of exercise and fresh air and also spectacular scenery. A walk around the park can be just the ticket to shift an awkward mood. Some ideas for other great places to walk can be found at <www.nationalparks.gov.uk> or <www.ramblers.org.uk/go-walking/find-a-walk-or-route.aspx>.

Take care of yourself: do check weather conditions and go appropriately dressed and equipped.

Gardening

Gardening is another activity, surging in popularity in recent years, from which many people gain health and well-being benefits. If you don't have your own garden and would like to look into it, some places have community gardens or community allotments where you can get involved alongside others. Contact your local council or allotment society for information. Or get more information from either the National Society of Allotment and Leisure Gardeners, <www.nsalg.org.uk>, or the Royal Horticultural Society, <www.rhs.org.uk>.

Waiting times for allotments can be quite long, but you may well find that people have a patch that they are willing to 'lend' to a co-worker – ask at your local site.

Learning and personal development

In Chapter 4 we looked at 'recovery colleges' or 'recovery academies'. We know that one of your mental five-a-day is to *keep learning*, but quite possibly you might not want to spend your leisure time thinking about yourself or your own well-being. It is possible to access other forms of learning for free or at minimal cost if you are on a low income, including learning for work skills development, learning for academic qualifications and learning for pleasure. Of course, learning can be informal and picked up from friends and family too – map reading, using office software, embroidery.

Work and home

Meaningful work that neither stresses you out nor makes you ill – and pays you enough to live on – sometimes feels like the Holy Grail of adult life. It is difficult enough to achieve when you are in the best of health. For women in particular the recent recession has been very harsh, with working mothers hit particularly hard by redundancies. This has had knock-on effects in terms of self-esteem, family life and financial security. In this context, for a person in recovery to find and hold on to work can seem overwhelming.

It is worth reflecting on how many people *in work* are in recovery too. The support organizations listed in the previous section are very good starting points for advice about work options. If you feel, for whatever reason, that you are not 'employable' – if, for example, your health condition means frequent medical appointments, if you have a criminal record or if you have caring commitments – the Fredericks Foundation can help you work out if self-employment might be a suitable option for you (see p. 74).

Home – finding a suitable one, keeping it, making it a good place for you – is central to a decent life. You may need assistance with this, and you may have to compromise. Your local benefits advice service will be able to advise whether you are entitled to financial help or social housing. If you have a mortgage, speak with your mortgage company if for any reason you are struggling to make payments: the guidance on how people should be treated in these circumstances has improved in recent years. If you have children you should be treated with particular respect and care. As circumstances change from time to time and place to place, get up-to-date advice from your CAB or preferred source of trusted support as soon as you need it. Home is a place in your heart and mind as well as the physical structure you live in. It's the place where you live, love and recover.

Maybe your motivation to deal with aspects of your recovery comes and goes. That is normal. Maybe it feels as if there is too much to tackle and not enough energy or help to do it all. That's normal too. You do not (and indeed cannot) do everything at once, so make a list of all the things that matter and prioritize – decide the order of importance for things and use that to guide what you do. Here is one way of organizing things in order of importance:[4]

1 Does it meet a fundamental human need (food, shelter, sleep)? Is it essential for your physical and mental health and survival?
2 Does it help to keep you safe and well?
3 Does it meet your need for human contact, love or conversation?

4 Does it make you feel good about yourself and the world?

5 Does it help to make you a better, more capable or more creative person?

There is not much point tackling item 5 if you have not got everything you need from item 1 in place.

It is easy to lose sight of the basics – looking after yourself and those who depend on you comes first. Get help, accept imperfection, be kind. Good luck.

Notes

Introduction

1 The Royal Society of Arts' pioneering Whole Person Recovery project. See <www.thersa.org/action-research-centre/reports/socialchange/whole-person-recovery>.

2 I.e. detain in hospital without the individual's agreement under the provisions of the Mental Health Act 1983. See <www.mind.org.uk/information-support/legal-rights/mental-health-act-the-mind-guide/about-the-mental-health-act/#.VFzrvfmsVV0 >.

1 Same as it ever was

1 Quoted by Rebecca Daddow and Steve Broome, *Whole Person Recovery: A user-centred systems approach to problem drug use* (London: RSA, 2010), p. 100

2 Daddow and Broome, *Whole Person Recovery*, p. 101

3 Abraham J. Twerski, *Addictive Thinking: Understanding self-deception* (Center City, MN: Hazelden, 1990)

4 Twerski, *Addictive Thinking*, p. 6

5 Twerski, *Addictive Thinking*, p. 41

6 Twerski, *Addictive Thinking*, p. 45

7 Twerski, *Addictive Thinking*, p. 49

8 Melody Beattie, *Codependent No More* (Center City, MN: Hazelden, 1992), p. 36

9 Twerski, *Addictive Thinking*, p. 49

10 Quoted by Miranda Critchley in her review of Michael Clune, *White Out* (Center City, MN: Hazelden, 2013), *London Review of Books*, vol. 36, no. 21, 6 November 2014

11 Stanton Peele, 'Addiction Myths', accessed online July 2014

12 Critchley, *London Review of Books*, 6 November 2014

13 There is more information about PAWS at <www.addictionsandrecovery.org/post-acute-withdrawal.htm>

14 Ruth Chandler, Simon Bradstreet and Mark Hayward, *Voicing Caregiver Experiences: Wellbeing and recovery narratives for caregivers* (Hove: Sussex Partnership NHS Foundation Trust and the Scottish Recovery Network, 2013)

15 Dave Mearns and Brian Thorne, *Person-Centred Counselling in Action*, 4th edn (London: Sage, 2013), p. 15

16 Daddow and Broome, *Whole Person Recovery*, p. 44

17 Daddow and Broome, *Whole Person Recovery*, p. 107

28 Catherine Amey, *Psychosis Through My Eyes* (Brentwood: Chipmunka Publishing, 2012), p. 39

2 Into the blue again

1 <www.drugscope.org.uk/Resources/Drugscope/Documents/PDF/Policy/MarcusreportICM.pdf>
2 Sussex Partnership NHS Foundation Trust, *Research* magazine, 2014:4, p. 12
3 <www.nhsconfed.org/resources/key-statistics-on-the-nhs>
4 <www.nice.org.uk/guidance/CG100/chapter/introduction>
5 <www.ibtimes.co.uk/mental-health-reduced-life-expectancy-nhs-reforms-450459>
6 <www.nhsconfed.org/resources/key-statistics-on-the-nhs>
7 Rebecca Daddow and Steve Broome, *Whole Person Recovery: A user-centred systems approach to problem drug use* (London: RSA, 2010), p. iv
8 *Diagnostic and Statistical Manual of Mental Disorders*, 5th edn (Arlington, VA: American Psychiatric Publishing, 2013)
9 <www.dsm5.org/Documents/Substance%20Use%20Disorder%20Fact%20Sheet.pdf>
10 <addictions.about.com/od/aboutaddiction/a/Dsm-5-Criteria-For-Substance-Use-Disorders.htm>
11 Joanne Neale, Sarah Nettleton and Lucy Pickering, *The Everyday Lives of Recovering Heroin Users* (London: RSA, 2012)
12 Neale, Nettleton and Pickering, *Everyday Lives*, p. 29
13 <www.prisonreformtrust.org.uk/Portals/0/Documents/Prisonthefacts.pdf>
14 <www.prisonreformtrust.org.uk/Portals/0/Documents/Prisonthefacts.pdf>
15 'June', 'Surviving Social Disadvantage: A Testimony to Courage', in Richard Worsley and Stephen Joseph, eds, *Person-Centred Practice: Case studies in positive psychology* (Ross-on-Wye: PCCS Books, 2007).
16 <www.nice.org.uk/guidance/cg115>. See also <www.nice.org.uk/guidance/cg51> on psycho-social care and drug detoxification
17 Daddow and Broome, *Whole Person Recovery*, p. 57
18 <www.drugscope.org.uk/Resources/Drugscope/Documents/PDF/Policy/MarcusreportICM.pdf>
19 J. Hoare and D. Moon, *Drug Misuse Declared: Findings from the 2009/2010 British Crime Survey* (London: Home Office, 2010)
20 Daddow and Broome, *Whole Person Recovery*, p. 3
21 Daddow and Broome, *Whole Person Recovery*, p. 57

3 Once in a lifetime

1 Rebecca Daddow and Steve Broome, *Whole Person Recovery: A user-centred systems approach to problem drug use* (London: RSA, 2010), p. 56
2 Types of anti-depressant medication. For more information about these, see <www.mind.org.uk/information-support/drugs-and-treatments/antidepressants/>
3 Daddow and Broome, *Whole Person Recovery*, p.115

4   My current favourite example is the pioneering availability of creative activities at NHS premises for people with long-term conditions, such as at GP Innovators of the Year, Brighton Health and Wellbeing Centre.

5   <www.rethink.org/diagnosis-treatment/treatment-and-support/assertive-outreach>

6   <http://www.rethink.org/diagnosis-treatment/treatment-and-support/assertive-outreach>

7   Daddow and Broome, *Whole Person Recovery*, p. 116

8   <www.mentalhealth.org.uk/help-information/mental-health-a-z/r/recovery/>

9   Sainsbury Centre for Mental Health, quoted in Daddow and Broome *Whole Person Recovery*, p. 8

10 For those wanting to read in more depth, see for example S. Patterson et al., *User Involvement in Efforts to Improve the Quality of Drug Misuse Services* (London: UK Department of Health, 2007); J. Fischer et al, *Drug User Involvement in Treatment Decisions* (York: Joseph Rowntree Foundation, 2007)

11 Daddow and Broome, *Whole Person Recovery*, p. 21

12 See e.g. <www.thefix.com/content/russell-brand-misguided-crusade-against-methadone-maintenance00228?page=all>

13 Joanne Neale, Sarah Nettleton and Lucy Pickering, *The Everyday Lives of Recovering Heroin Users* (London: RSA, 2012), p. 34

14 Neale, Nettleton and Pickering, *Everyday Lives*, p. 43

15 See <www.aa.org/pages/en_US/read-the-big-book-and-twelve-steps-and-twelve-traditions>.

16 See for example Sigmund Freud, *The Interpretation of Dreams* (Harmondsworth: Penguin, 1976), p. 118

17 Rogers himself in 1961 wrote a highly readable and accessible introduction to his ideas, *On Becoming a Person: A therapist's view of psychotherapy* (London: Constable, 1967)

18 Neale, Nettleton and Pickering, *Everyday Lives*, p. 89

19 Interviewee, *Whole Person Recovery*, p. 55

20 Dave Mearns and Brian Thorne, *Person-Centred Counselling in Action*, 4th edn (London: Sage, 2013)

21 Mearns and Thorne, *Person-Centred Counselling*, p. 101

22 Daddow and Broome, *Whole Person Recovery*, p.58

23 Workshop participants at a training day facilitated by the author, Brighton, May 2014

24 Decca Aitkenhead, 'Liar, Addict, Reformed Man?', *Guardian Weekend* magazine, 3 January 2015, p. 30

25 Audio and video of the talk he gave in London in 2011 can be found at <www.thersa.org/events/audio-and-past-events/2011/addiction-what-to-do-when-everything-else-has-failed>.

26

27 Bruce Alexander, *The Globalization of Addiction: A study in poverty of the spirit*, Introduction (Oxford: Oxford University Press, 2008).

4 It's not yesterday any more

1 Georgia W., *Don't Let the Bastards Grind You Down: 50 things every alcoholic and addict in early recovery should know* (Denver, CO: Ornery Tiger Press, 2008)
2 Georgia W., *Don't Let the Bastards*, p. 29
3 Georgia W., *Don't Let the Bastards*, p. 45
4
5 <lithgow-schmidt.dk/sherry-arnstein/ladder-of-citizen-participation. html>

5 Other recovery tools

1 <http://www.alcohollearningcentre.org.uk/_library/Alcohol_ Outcomes_Star_user_Guide.pdf>
2 <www.outcomesstar.org.uk/storage/star-guide-previews/mental-health-recovery-star/Recovery-Star-User-Guide-3rd-Ed-preview.pdf>
3 Rebecca Daddow and Steve Broome, *Whole Person Recovery: A user-centred systems approach to problem drug use* (London: RSA, 2010), p. 109
4 <www.recovery.org/topics/alcoholics-anonymous-12-step/>
5 See
6 <www.grow.org.au/grow-program/>
7 <www.smartrecovery.org/resources/library/Articles_and_Essays/ Additional_Articles/abstinence_vs_moderation.htm>
8 <www.ihra.net/what-is-harm-reduction>
9 <www.nhs.uk/Conditions/stress-anxiety-depression/Pages/improve-mental-wellbeing.aspx#Sarah>
10 <www.nhs.uk/Conditions/stress-anxiety-depression/Pages/improve-mental-wellbeing.aspx#Evidence>
11 <www.gmw.nhs.uk/recovery>
12 Howard Gardner, *Frames of Mind: The theory of multiple intelligences* (New York: Basic Books, 1983) and *Multiple Intelligences* (New York: Basic Books, 1993, revised edn 2006)
13 Maya Angelou, *Wouldn't Take Nothing For My Journey Now* (New York: Random House, 1993), p. 138
14 Adapted from <www.mentalhealth.org.uk/help-information/mental-health-a-z/r/recovery/>
15 Daddow and Broome, *Whole Person Recovery*, p. 104
16 Daddow and Broome, *Whole Person Recovery*, p. 105
17 Daddow and Broome, *Whole Person Recovery*, p. 106
18 Daddow and Broome, *Whole Person Recovery*, p. 109
19 Daddow and Broome, *Whole Person Recovery*, p. 109
20 Johann Hari, *Guardian Weekend* magazine, 3 January 2015, p. 31
21 Daddow and Broome, *Whole Person Recovery*, p. 100
22 <www.lrb.co.uk/v36/n21/miranda-critchley/dont-be-dull>
23 Decca Aitkenhead, 'Liar, Addict, Reformed Man?', *Guardian Weekend* magazine, 3 January 2015, p. 30

24 Quoted by Miranda Critchley in her review of Michael Clune, *White Out* (Center City, MN: Hazelden, 2013), *London Review of Books*, vol. 36, no. 21, 6 November 2014

25 Brendan Kennelly, from 'Begin', in *Familiar Strangers: New and selected poems 1960–2004* (Hexham: Bloodaxe Books, 2004)

Helpful organizations

1 <www.cnwl.nhs.uk/services/mental-health-services/rehabilitation/inpatient-rehabilitation>

Other resources for recovery

1 See for example <www.liv.ac.uk/psychology-health-and-society/research/reading-literature-and-society/research-projects/>

2 See <readingagency.org.uk/adults/quick-guides/reading-well/>

3 <network.youthmusic.org.uk/learning/blogs/rhythmix/mitch-winehouse-present-rhythmix-funding-and-speak-surrey-music-hub-conferen>

4 Based on Maslow's Hierarchy of Needs, a tool commonly used in psychology, e.g. at <www.simplypsychology.org/maslow.html>

References

How do you summarize a life's reading? For me, books were my salvation, my escape, my education, my route map to the future. Having grown up on a council estate in what policy-makers and social workers these days may refer to as a 'troubled family', the likelihood of my ending up in trouble and addiction was far greater than of going to Cambridge University to study literature, which is what actually happened. Reading was the secret – if you hadn't guessed already. I have made use of that a great deal in my involvement in recovery work, but I could not possibly list all the books I have found helpful or beneficial. So this list is just of those I have used most directly in this handbook.

Al-Anon, *Alcoholism: A Merry-Go-Round Named Denial*, Virginia Beach, VA: Al Anon, 1969

Alcoholics Anonymous, *The Big Book*, AA, 1932

Alexander, Bruce, *The Globalization of Addiction: A study in poverty of the spirit*, Oxford: Oxford University Press, 2008

Amey, Catherine, *Psychosis Through My Eyes*, Brentwood: Chipmunka Publishing, 2012

Angelou, Maya, *Wouldn't Take Nothing For My Journey Now*, New York: Random House, 1993

Barnard, Marina, *Drug Addiction and Families*, London: Jessica Kingsley, 2006

Beattie, Melody, *Codependent No More*, Center City, MN: Hazelden, 1992

Benjamin, Jessica, *The Bonds of Love: Psychoanalysis, feminism, and the problem of domination*, London: Virago, 1990

Best, David, *Addiction Recovery: A handbook – a movement for social change and personal growth in the UK*, Amazon Kindle ebook, 2012

Bifulco, Antonia and Moran, Patricia, *Wednesday's Child: Research into women's experience of neglect and abuse in childhood, and adult depression*, London: Routledge, 1998

Cantopher, Tim, *Depressive Illness: The curse of the strong*, London: Sheldon Press, 2003

Chandler, Ruth, Bradstreet, Simon and Hayward, Mark, *Voicing Caregiver Experiences: Wellbeing and recovery narratives for caregivers*, Hove: Sussex Partnership NHS Foundation Trust, 2014

Cline, Sally and Spender, Dale, *Reflecting Men at Twice Their Natural Size: Why women work at making men feel good*, Glasgow: Fontana, 1987

Clune, Michael, *White Out: The secret life of heroin*, Center City, MN: Hazelden, 2014

Cooper, Mick, *Essential Research Findings in Counselling and Psychotherapy*, London: Sage/BACP, 2008

Covey, Stephen R., *Seven Habits of Highly Effective People*, Simon and Schuster, 1989

Daddow, Rebecca and Broome, Steve, *Whole Person Recovery: A user-centred systems approach to problem drug use*, London: Royal Society of Arts, 2010

Dryden, Windy and Feltham, Colin, eds, *Psychotherapy and Its Discontents*, Buckingham: Open University Press, 1992

Freud, Sigmund, *The Interpretation of Dreams*, Harmondsworth: Penguin, 1976

Gardner, Howard, *Frames of Mind: The theory of multiple intelligences*, New York: Basic Books, 1983

Gratch, Alon, *If Men Could Talk . . . This is what they would say*, New York: Little, Brown, 2001

Hoare, J. and Moon, D., *Drug Misuse Declared: Findings from the 2009/2010 British Crime Survey*, London: Home Office, 2010

Howe, David, *On Being a Client*, London: Sage, 1993

Jung, Carl, and von Franz, M. L., eds, *Man and His Symbols*, London: Aldus Books, 1964

McGregor, Jane and McGregor, Tim, *The Empathy Trap: Understanding anti-social personalities*, London: Sheldon Press, 2013

Mearns, David and Thorne, Brian, *Person-Centred Counselling in Action*, 4th edn, London: Sage, 2013

Miller, Alice, *The Untouched Key: Tracing childhood trauma in creativity and destructiveness*, London: Virago, 1990

Milner, Marion, *A Life of One's Own*, London: Virago, 1986

Neale, Joanne, Nettleton, Sarah and Pickering, Lucy, *The Everyday Lives of Recovering Heroin Users*, London: Royal Society of Arts, 2012

Porter, Roy, *Mind-Forg'd Manacles: A history of madness in England from the Restoration to the Regency*, London: Athlone Press, 1987

Porter, Roy, *The Greatest Benefit to Mankind: A medical history of humanity from antiquity to the present*, London: HarperCollins, 1997

Roberts, Marcus, *What Does the Public Really Think About Drug Addiction and Its Treatment?*, London: Drugscope, 2009

Rogers, Carl R., *On Becoming a Person: A therapist's view of psychotherapy*, London: Constable, 1967

Triangle/Mental Health Providers Forum, *Recovery Star Users Guide*, 3rd edn, www.outcomesstar.org.uk

Trower, Peter et al., *Cognitive Behavioural Counselling in Action*, 2nd edn, London: Sage, 2011

Twerski, Abraham J., *Addictive Thinking: Understanding self-deception*, Center City, MN: Hazelden, 1990

W., Georgia, *Don't Let the Bastards Grind You Down*, Denver, CO: Ornery Tiger Press, 2009

Ward, Deborah, *Overcoming Fear with Mindfulness*, London: Sheldon Press, 2013

Wilson, John, *Supporting People Through Loss and Grief: An introduction for counsellors and other caring practitioners*, London: Jessica Kingsley, 2014

Worsley, Richard and Joseph, Stephen, *Person-Centred Practice: Case studies in positive psychology*, Ross-on-Wye: PCCS Books, 2007

Index

Page numbers in **bold** print indicate principal entries.